Assessing the Youthful Offender

Issues and Techniques

Forensic Psychiatry and Psychology Library

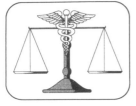

Series Editor
Seymour Halleck
The University of North Carolina
Chapel Hill, North Carolina

Assessing the Youthful Offender
Issues and Techniques
Robert D. Hoge and D. A. Andrews

A Continuation Order Plan is available for this series. A continuation order will bring delivery of each new volume immediately upon publication. Volumes are billed only upon actual shipment. For further information please contact the publisher.

Assessing the Youthful Offender

Issues and Techniques

Robert D. Hoge

and

D. A. Andrews

Carleton University
Ottawa, Ontario, Canada

Plenum Press • New York and London

Library of Congress Cataloging-in-Publication Data

Hoge, Robert D.
    Assessing the youthful offender : issues and techniques / Robert
D. Hoge and D.A. Andrews.
      p.   ;cm. -- (Forensic psychiatry and psychology library)
    Includes bibliographical references and index.
    ISBN 0-306-45466-1. -- ISBN 0-306-45467-X (pbk.)
      1. Juvenile delinquents--Psychological testing.
    2. Psychodiagnostics. 3. Criminal psychology. 4. Forensic
    psychiatry. 5. Juvenile delinquency--Psychological aspects.
    6. Social work with juvenile delinquents.   I. Andrews, D. A.
    (Donald Arthur), 1941-   . II. Title. III. Series.
    HV6080.H58 1996
    364.3'6--dc21   96-39453
                                                               CIP

ISBN 0-306-45466-1 (Hardbound)
ISBN 0-306-45467-X (Paperback)

© 1996 Plenum Press, New York
A Division of Plenum Publishing Corporation
233 Spring Street, New York, N. Y. 10013

Printed in the United States of America

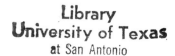

Foreword

Our society's preoccupation with crime and fear of crime appears to have shifted its focus to the juvenile offender. Both electronic and print media continuously warn us that juvenile offenders are increasingly younger and more virulent. The demographics of our population suggest that there will only be more juvenile offenders to fear in the near future.

All of these concerns arise in a social climate that is characterized by an ever-increasing demand for stronger retributive measures against the offender. The belief that only harsh justice will protect us from the ravages of juveniles has become dominant. Increasingly, perceptions and politics, rather than scientific data, dominate policy making with regard to youthful offenders.

In *Assessing the Youthful Offender: Issues and Techniques*, Robert D. Hoge and D. A. Andrews make a restrained, rational, and ultimately persuasive argument for the use of standardized psychological assessments in the effective management of youth within juvenile justice systems. They clarify how what we already know about the cause and management of youthful criminal activity can be incorporated into standardized testing and that the information obtained from testing can improve the administration of criminal justice. Moreover, this information is useful whatever the theoretical biases of those who administer the justice system. The efficiency of policies of either retribution, deterrence, or rehabilitation is only enhanced by reliance on data.

The authors have presented an understandable and highly readable description of current theories of criminal justice as well as a description of the state-of-the-art of modern standardized psychological assessment. Those who are familiar with the subject matter will find that this book helps them conceptualize the issues of criminal justice more clearly. Readers less familiar with the material will expand their knowledge in a quick and painless way. This book should be read by anyone who works in the criminal justice system, whatever his or her professional biases might be. It is a powerful reminder that there is a science of criminology which will ultimately benefit a society that is willing to use it.

Seymour Halleck
Series Editor

Preface

The primary goal of this volume is to show how standardized psychological assessments can improve the management of youth within juvenile justice systems. The volume developed out of two observations we have made through our interactions with individuals involved in youth justice systems and our research in this area. First, there is often a misunderstanding about the potential contributions of psychological assessments to the processing of the youthful offender. This misunderstanding, which exists at all levels of the judicial system, applies to both the strengths and the weaknesses of psychological assessments. Second, impressive advances are being made in the development and application of psychological assessments, many of which have relevance to juvenile justice systems.

The volume is also based on a set of assumptions we have formed from contemporary theoretical and empirical literature regarding the processing of youthful offenders. Although these assumptions are developed in detail in the volume, we will present them in outline form here.

First, we assume that decisions made about the youth within the justice system are always based on inferences or judgments about them or their circumstances. These judgments incorporate a broad range of variables relating to circumstances of the criminal act; the youths' mental, emotional, and behavioral functioning; their attitudes and values; and their family and community situation.

A second assumption is that these inferences and judgments are often made in an informal and unsystematic manner; that is, they are often formed by juvenile justice system personnel functioning with broad discretionary powers and limited procedural guidance. This often results in invalid and inconsistent judgments about youths, which in turn produces inappropriate and inequitable decisions.

Our third assumption is that the quality of inferences and judgments about the youth and the decisions based on them can be improved through the use of standardized psychological assessments. Later we discuss in some detail the advantages of using such assessments but will note here our two major arguments. First, the use of standardized psychological assessments with demonstrable reliability and validity levels can improve the quality of the judgments and inferences made about the youth. Second, the use of these assessments may encourage a consistent treatment of offenders across the system.

The volume is directed at four audiences. The first includes mental health practitioners involved in the conduct and interpretation of assessments of young offenders. This group comprises primarily psychologists, but those in other professional groups, including psychiatrists, social workers, and educators, are sometimes involved as well. The volume is designed to inform these professionals about the most recent developments in the assessment area relevant to forensic decision making. The second group includes probation officers, youth care workers, correctional officers, and other frontline workers. These individuals are sometimes involved in collecting and utilizing psychological assessments, and as we will see, there are increasing efforts to develop assessment tools appropriate for their use. The volume should help familiarize these individuals with the role of psychological assessments. The third group includes judicial personnel—judges and lawyers in particular—who are sometimes required to utilize psychological assessments. The discussions of the role of psychological assessments in forensic decision making in Chapters 1, 2, 3, and 8 are particularly relevant to this group. The final group includes criminologists, psychologists, and others who are involved in research and evaluation activities within juvenile justice systems. The volume informs them about the latest advances in assessment tools and identifies areas in which continued research efforts are required.

The volume is organized as follows: Chapter 1 contains an overview of the major models of juvenile justice and the various theoretical positions regarding the causes of youth crime. Chapter 2 then provides a discussion of the decision-making process as it occurs in juvenile justice systems. This chapter includes an outline of the major types of forensic decisions and the various categories of judgments underlying them. Chapter 3 provides a general discussion of the role of psychological assessments in juvenile justice systems and includes a review of the various potential strengths and weaknesses of using psychological assessments in forensic decision making and a discussion of the bases for evaluating psychological measures.

The following four chapters contain reviews of different types of psychological assessment tools appropriate for the juvenile justice system: aptitude and achievement tests (Chapter 4); measures of personality, behavior, and attitudes (Chapter 5); measures of environmental factors (Chapter 6); and diagnostic and classification systems (Chapter 7). Each chapter contains a general discussion of the different types of measures and their relevance to decisions made about youth within judicial systems. We also identify examples of the various types of measures; in selecting examples, we have generally identified measures and procedures that are the subject of current clinical and research activity.

It may also be useful to provide a comment on our views of the role of psychological assessments in forensic decision making and of optimal approaches to dealing with youth crime. Our discussion in Chapter 1 reflects the fact that there is a considerable difference of opinion regarding the treatment of youth crime. The positions range from the very punitive Crime Control Model to child-focused orientations directed at identifying and serving specific needs of youthful offenders. We feel that standardized psychological assessments, to the extent that they improve the validity of information collected about the client and encourage consistent treatment of clients, have a positive role to play no matter what type of orientation underlies the system. On the other hand, and as we make clear in Chapter 1, we favor a particular approach to dealing with youthful offenders, one that is best characterized as reflecting a child welfare and rehabilitative focus. The reader is advised to keep this orientation in mind in considering our treatment of the volume's subject matter.

A number of organizations and individuals have made valuable contributions to the preparation of this volume, and we would like to acknowledge that assistance. Our research with children and adolescents has been supported by funds from the Ontario Ministry of Community and Social Services, Health Canada's Strategic Fund for Children's Mental Health, and Carleton University. Earlier drafts of some chapters of the book were read by Ray Corrado, Robert Knights, Lynda Robertson, David Simourd, and Clare Stoddard; we are very grateful for their valuable comments and suggestions. Marlo Gal also provided useful help in the preparation of the manuscript. Finally, we wish to acknowledge with gratitude the encouragement and support provided by friends, colleagues, and, in particular, our families throughout the preparation of this volume.

Contents

1. **Conceptual and Theoretical Background** 1

    1. Models of Juvenile Justice 2
        1.1. Child Welfare Model 4
        1.2. Corporatist Model 4
        1.3. Modified Justice Model 5
        1.4. Justice Model 5
        1.5. Crime Control Model 6
        1.6. Purposes of Judicial Dispositions 6
    2. Theories of Delinquency 7
    3. A Contemporary Psychological Perspective 8

2. **Decision Making within Juvenile Justice Systems** 15

    1. Areas of Forensic Decision Making 15
        1.1. Police Investigation/Processing 16
        1.2. Intake/Preadjudicatory Processing 17
        1.3. Adjudication 17
        1.4. Disposition 18
    2. Judgments about the Youth and Their Circumstances 18
        2.1. Seriousness of Offense 19
        2.2. Aggravating and Mitigating Factors 20
        2.3. Mental Status/Maturity 21
        2.4. Risk Level 21
        2.5. Criminogenic Need 22
        2.6. Responsivity and Amenability to Treatment 23
    3. Decision-Making Processes 24

3. **The Role of Psychological Assessments in the Juvenile Justice Decision Process** 29

    1. Major Types of Instruments and Procedures 29
    2. Evaluating Forensic Assessments 30
        2.1. Professional Standards 31
        2.2. Evaluation Terminology 32
    3. Potential Strengths of Standardized Psychological Assessments .. 38

4. Potential Drawbacks of Psychological Assessments 39
5. Organization of the Review 41

4. Assessing Aptitudes and Achievement Levels **43**

1. Aptitude Assessment Measures 43
   1.1. Tests of General Cognitive Ability 43
   1.2. Measures of Specific Aptitudes 47
   1.3. Neuropsychological Assessments 48
   1.4. Vocational Aptitude and Interest Tests 49
2. Measures of Academic Achievement 50
3. The Role of Aptitude and Achievement Measures in Juvenile
   Justice Systems 51

5. Assessing Personality, Attitudes, and Behaviors **55**

1. Personality Tests 55
2. Behavioral Ratings and Checklists 59
   2.1. Measures of Social and Emotional Competence and
        Pathology 59
   2.2. Measures of Antisocial and Self-Destructive Behaviors 60
   2.3. Measures of Adaptive Functioning 61
3. Interview Schedules 62
4. Other Types of Personality and Behavioral Measures 64
5. Measures of Attitudes, Values, and Beliefs 64
6. The Role of Personality, Behavioral, and Attitudinal Measures in
   Juvenile Justice Systems 65

6. Assessing Environmental Factors **69**

1. Measures of Family Functioning and Parenting 70
2. Measures of School Performance and Adjustment 72
3. Measures of Peer Group Associations 73
4. Measures of Correctional and Therapeutic Environments 74
5. The Role of Environmental Assessments in Juvenile Justice
   Systems 75

7. Diagnostic and Classification Systems **79**

1. Personality-Based Diagnostic Systems 79
   1.1. *Diagnostic and Statistical Manual of Mental Disorders,*
        Fourth Edition (DSM-IV) 80
   1.2. The Minnesota Multiphasic Personality Inventory 81
   1.3. The Interpersonal Maturity Level Classification System 82
   1.4. The Conceptual Level Matching Model (CLMM) 83
2. Behaviorally Based Systems 84

3. Offense-Based Risk Systems 84
4. Broad-Based Risk and Risk/Need Instruments 87
    4.1. The Wisconsin Juvenile Probation and Aftercare Assessment
        Form 87
    4.2. The Arizona Juvenile Risk Assessment Form 88
    4.3. The Firesetting Risk Interview 88
    4.4. The Psychopathy Checklist–Revised (PCL-R) 88
    4.5. The Youth Level of Service/Case Management Inventory
        (YLS/CMI) 90
5. Other Diagnostic Instruments 92
6. The Role of Diagnostic and Classification Systems in Juvenile
   Justice Systems 93
    6.1. Personality- and Behaviorally Based Systems 93
    6.2. Offense-Based Risk Systems 94
    6.3. Broad-Based Risk and Risk/Need Systems 94

8. Conclusions and Recommendations **97**

1. Positive Contributions of the Assessments 97
    1.1. Availability of Tools 97
    1.2. Consistency 98
    1.3. Explicitness of Constructs 98
    1.4. Access to Substantive Findings 99
    1.5. Evaluation Methodology 100
    1.6. System Efficiency 100
2. Recommendations for Practitioners 100
    2.1. The Role of Professional Expertise 101
    2.2. Selection of Instruments 102
3. Research Recommendations 105
    3.1. Criminological Processes 106
    3.2. Construct Development 107
    3.3. Instrument Development 108
4. Concluding Comments 109

**Appendix 1: Instruments and Procedures Identified in This
Volume** **111**

Appendix 2: Addresses of Major Test Publishers **115**

References **117**

Author Index **129**

Subject Index **133**

Assessing the Youthful Offender

Issues and Techniques

Chapter 1 ☐

Conceptual and Theoretical Background

The goal of this volume is to show how standardized psychological assessments can be used to enhance the quality of decisions made about young people in the juvenile justice system. Standardized psychological assessments are those with fixed formats and for which psychometric data are available. They include individual assessment instruments, such as the Minnesota Multiphasic Inventory (MMPI), as well as more comprehensive assessment procedures, such as the Conceptual Level Matching Model. We will discuss the nature of these assessments in more detail in later chapters.

Our analysis of the decision process in the justice context is based on the framework developed by Gottfredson and Gottfredson (1988). Within this model, judicial and quasijudicial decisions are viewed as reflecting choices among alternative courses of action, with the choices based on (1) the acceptance of certain goals, (2) assumptions about the way in which the various alternative courses of action relate to those goals, (3) judgments about the client bearing on those assumptions, and (4) a final choice among the alternatives.

To illustrate, a judge's decision to sentence a young person to a period of secure custody may reflect (1) the goal of deterring that young person from committing future crimes; (2) an assumption that a young person who has committed a serious crime, who is from a dysfunctional home environment, and who shows little remorse for the crime is most likely to be deterred from future criminal activity through a period of incarceration; and (3) inferences that this particular young person exhibits the conditions reflected in the assumption.

Three sources of invalid or inappropriate decisions may be identified in this framework. The first relates to the assumptions made about the alternative courses of action. These may be erroneous, and the chosen course of action may not, in fact, lead to the desired goal. It is possible, for example, that the experience of secure custody does not act as a deterrent for future criminal activity in the case of a young person exhibiting the conditions described above. We feel that psychological and criminological research has much to contribute to the evaluation of the assumptions underlying decisions within the juvenile justice system, but that issue is not the major concern of this work.

The second source of inappropriate decisions involves the use of invalid inferences or judgments about the young person within the decision process. Choices among alternative courses of action are always based on inferences or judgments about the young person, and these, in turn, are based on information about the client collected from interviews, observations, file information, court records, and other such sources. Where this information is incorrect, irrelevant, or processed inappropriately, invalid inferences may be produced, and these, in turn, may lead to inappropriate choices among the alternative courses of action. To illustrate with the above example, if the judge's inferences about the home environment and the youth's level of remorse are incorrect, then the decision to refer the youth to custody may be inappropriate.

The third source of inappropriate or invalid decisions within this framework arises from the inconsistent application of decision rules within systems. This situation usually arises when personnel within a system are afforded considerable decision-making discretion and when they embrace different goals and assumptions. To return to the example, other judges within the system may make different assumptions about the role of custody and, hence, may apply different decision rules in their disposition decisions.

Our primary concern is with the latter two sources of inappropriate decisions, and the goal of this volume is to demonstrate that standardized psychological assessment instruments and procedures can play a positive role in the judicial decision-making process by improving the collection and utilization of information about clients and thus contribute to more effective decisions about the young person.

It is important to recognize that there are a number of alternative models of juvenile justice, and those models are based on several conflicting theories of the causes of youth crime. We believe that standardized psychological assessments have a role to play in juvenile justice systems regardless of models. On the other hand, the role of these assessments varies somewhat with the focus of the system, and we next turn to an outline of the major models of juvenile justice and theories of youth crime as a background to our discussion of psychological assessments. We conclude the chapter with a discussion of a contemporary perspective regarding the causes and treatment of youth crime.

1. □ Models of Juvenile Justice

Corrado (1992) has identified five broad models of juvenile justice (see Figure 1.1), and, although these models exist nowhere in a pure form, they are useful ways of viewing some philosophically different approaches to the treatment of the youthful offender. These models differ in terms of the goals they adopt for the judicial process and the assumptions they make regarding the best means of achieving those goals. The models also differ, as we will see, in the implications they have for the assessment of the youthful offender.

Characteristics	Welfare[1,2] *Focus on offender*	Corporatism[1]	Modified Justice	Justice[1]	Crime Control[2] *Focus on protection of society*
General features	Informality; Generic referrals; Individualized sentencing; Indeterminate sentencing	Administrative decision making; Offending; Diversion from court/custody programs; Alternative to care/custody programs	Due process informality; Criminal offenses; Bifurcation: soft offenders diverted, hard offenders punished; Determinate sentences	Due process; Criminal offenses; Least restrictive alternative; Determinate sentences	Due process/discretion; Offending/status offenses; Punishment; Determinate sentences
Key personnel	Childcare experts	Juvenile justice specialists	Lawyers/childcase experts	Lawyers	Lawyers/criminal justice actors
Key agency	Social work	Interagency structure	Law/social work	Law	Law
Tasks	Diagnosis	Systems intervention	Diagnosis/punishment	Punishment	Incarceration/punishment
Understanding of client behavior	Pathology/environmentally determined	Unsocialized	Diminished individual responsibility	Individual responsibility	Responsibility/accountability
Purpose of intervention	Provide treatment (parens patriae)	Retrain	Sanction behavior/provide treatment	Sanction behavior	Protection of society/retribution/deterrence
Objectives	Respond to individual needs/rehabilitation	Implementation of policy	Respect individual rights/respond to "special" needs	Respect individual rights/punish	Order maintenance

[1]Pratt, "Corporatism: The Third Model of Juvenile Justice (1989) 29(3) *Br. J.C.* pp. 236–53.
[2]Reid and Reitsma-Street, "Assumptions and Implications of New Canadian Legislation for Young Offenders" (1984) 17(1) *C.C.F.* pp. 334–52.
Source: Corrado (1992). Copyright © Butterworths Canada Ltd., 1992. All rights reserved. Reprinted by permission of Harcourt Brace & Company, Canada, Limited.

Figure 1.1. □ Continuum of juvenile justice models.

1.1. ☐ Child Welfare Model

The Child Welfare Model served as the primary guide to the treatment of the youthful offender in the Canadian, American, and British juvenile justice systems from around the turn of the century to recent years. There have been rather significant shifts away from this position in these systems over the recent past, although it continues to exert an influence.

The principal objectives within this approach focus on the enhancement of the functioning of the young person, with the ultimate goal of turning them away from a life of crime toward a productive and prosocial lifestyle. The approach has also generally reflected a doctrine of *parens patriae*, the concept that, under some circumstances, the state has the right to assume responsibility for the well-being of the young person.

The key assumptions within this approach are that sanctioning and punishment activities should play little role in the management of the youthful offender. Rather, it is assumed that interventions that draw on medical, psychological, educational, or social work techniques and are directed toward the youth and/or his or her family or community situation will have the desired rehabilitative effects. It must be recognized, though, that the specific assumptions about desirable courses of action depend on more fundamental assumptions about the causes of youthful criminal activity. We will review the various theoretical positions relevant to this model in the next section and simply note here that there exists a considerable range of views within this model about the direction that rehabilitation efforts should take.

The demands made on the assessment process within this approach reflect its focus on the needs of the individual offender. The required assessments involve diagnoses of the situational and individual factors that are directly related to the criminal activity. These assessments may be viewed as critical to the process of making rational choices among alternative rehabilitative strategies. In general, then, a broad role exists for psychological assessments within this type of model.

1.2. ☐ Corporatist Model

The Corporatist Model has been described by Corrado (1992), Corrado and Turnbull (1992), and Pratt (1989) as representative of the juvenile justice system that has most recently evolved in England and Wales; it is also in some respects descriptive of the system observed in the Canadian province of Quebec (Le Blanc & Beaumont, 1992). This model shares with the child welfare approach an emphasis on interventions aimed at the specific needs of the youthful offender, but it departs from that model by endeavoring to move the interventions out of the criminal justice system and into the wider network of social agencies dealing with children and families:

> The Corporatist Model emphasizes not the role of police (according to the Crime Control Model), nor the role of lawyers (according to the Justice Model), nor the role of social workers and other helping professions (according to the Welfare Model), but rather the roles of *all* of these groups acting in an interagency structure which efficiently diverts minor offenders, requires less serious property offenders and violent offenders to participate in attendance programs and sentences the few serious offenders to custodial institutions. (Corrado & Turnbull, 1992, p. 77)

Perhaps the most desirable feature of the model is represented in its goal of integrating all services for at-risk youths.

This model makes demands on assessment activities that are similar to those of the Child Welfare Model; that is, it calls for a broad assessment of all needs of the youth and an effort to match those needs with available services. This involves, then, assessing not only judicially relevant factors (e.g., seriousness of the crime, prior history of offending), but also the social, emotional, and educational needs of the young person.

1.3. □ Modified Justice Model

The Modified Justice Model is described by Corrado and Markwart (1992) and Corrado and Turnbull (1992) as representative of the type of juvenile justice system that has evolved in most jurisdictions in the United States and Canada over the past few years. The model incorporates both the treatment/rehabilitation focus of the Child Welfare Model and the concern for sanctioning and civil rights of the Justice Model. The trend in United States jurisdictions in particular has been toward the sanctioning component of the model, but in most cases some elements of a rehabilitation focus have been retained.

The demands on assessment services are as heavy in this type of system as in either of the previous two discussed here. Not only is there a requirement for information about the social and emotional needs of the youth, but data regarding criminogenic circumstances are also required as a basis for determining sanctions.

1.4. □ Justice Model

In the Justice Model, the focus shifts from a concern for the needs of the individual offender toward the criminal act and the appropriate legal responses to that act. The principal goals within this approach are to ensure that the civil or procedural rights of the youth are protected and that a disposition appropriate to the crime is established. Rehabilitative efforts are not excluded from consideration in this approach, but they are secondary to the concern for sanctioning the criminal act.

It should be noted that there is some debate within this model regarding the appropriate basis for criminal sanctions. In one case a utilitarian position is adopted: Punishment is designed primarily to reduce the likelihood that the young person will commit future crimes. The other position within the model reflects a purely punishment orientation. One form of the latter is the just deserts philosophy, which asserts that retribution is the only basis for punishment and that the severity of the sanction should reflect only the seriousness of the crime and the culpability of the offender.

In general, psychological assessments play a more limited role in the Justice Model than in the three previously described. The focus in this model is primarily on the criminal act, and, hence, assessments usually involve attention to issues of the seriousness of the act and the culpability of the offender. However, there are circumstances where other legally mandated assessments may be required; these assessments may relate to aggravating and mitigating factors, mental competency, or risk for future criminal activity.

1.5. □ Crime Control Model

The Crime Control Model described by Corrado and Markwart (1992) shares with the Justice Model a concern with legal processing and an emphasis on the legal sanctioning of the criminal act, but it views legal interventions as primarily designed to incapacitate or punish the offender and serve as a general deterrence for future criminal activities. Protection of society constitutes the primary goal of this approach. Police, prosecutors, and judges typically play the primary role in systems governed by this type of model.

Criminal sanctions involving incarceration are the preferred course of action within this model for career and/or violent offenders, although for minor or first offenses diversion or other types of alternatives might be considered. This model generally gives little weight to rehabilitation efforts. One could point to the youth justice system in Singapore as an example of this model; what might be considered as minor offenses elsewhere are considered major there and are sometimes dealt with through severe punishment.

Assessment activities within this model generally focus on judgments about the severity of the offense and risk for future criminal activity. As we will see, the assessment of risk, while presenting particular difficulties, is one area of forensic assessment in which significant advances are being made.

1.6. □ Purposes of Judicial Dispositions

It is clear from the discussion so far that there are conflicting assumptions about the goals of judicial dispositions within these alternative models. Since these have rather direct implications for assessment activities, we have summarized them in Table 1.1. The specific deterrence, general deterrence, retributive, and just deserts orientations are primarily relevant to the Justice and Crime Control models. They also, as we have seen, make minimal demands on assessment activities. The

Table 1.1. □ **Outline of the Major Purposes of Judicial Dispositions**

Purpose	Description
Specific deterence	Reduce reoffending on the part of the individual through the application of an appropriate punishment
General deterrence	Reduce the chances of offending on the part of those who observe the punishment of offeners
Incapacitation	Reduce reoffending during the period of the penalty through controls such as custody
Retribution	Cause offenders to suffer a punishment proportionate to harm suffered by their victim
Just desserts	Impose a punishment on the offender proportionate to the severity of their offense
Restoration	Restore balance in the community through mediation/conflict resolution and/or the impositions of fines, services, or other such forms of restitution
Rehabilitation	Reduce the chances of reoffending by targeting the criminogenic needs of the youth through human services

incapacitation, restoration, and rehabilitative orientations are most prominent in the Child Welfare, Corporatism, and Modified Justice models, and these orientations require more intensive assessments. We will pursue this issue in more detail in later chapters.

2. □ Theories of Delinquency

Implicit within each of the models discussed in this chapter are various theories of delinquency, that is, sets of assumptions and propositions regarding the causes of delinquent activity and the best means of addressing the problem. For example, the Justice Model is based on what is sometimes referred to as the neoclassical theory of crime; this is the theory that criminal acts are a product of conscious self-serving motives and that individuals will be discouraged from criminal activities through threats of punishment that outweigh the benefits of the action. The Child Welfare Model, on the other hand, locates the multiple causes of antisocial behavior within the family/personality/behavioral dynamics of individuals and/or their environment. It assumes that delinquency can best be addressed by dealing with these underlying causes.

It is also important to note, however, that conflicting theories are sometimes represented in the same model. For example, there has long been a conflict within the Child Welfare Model over a focus on psychological causation (flowing from a psychodynamic type of theory) or on social/economic causation (flowing, for example, from anomie theory). This conflict, as we will see, has important implications for assessment and intervention activities.

Table 1.2 provides an outline of the major theoretical positions regarding criminal behavior. Detailed discussions of those positions may be found in Akers (1994), Andrews and Bonta (1994), and Morris and Giller (1987), and a review of those discussions reveals the breadth and vitality of efforts to develop a theoretical understanding of the causes of criminal activity in young people. One criticism of these traditional theories, however, concerns their tendency to focus on one level of analysis, be it social forces, interpersonal dynamics, or psychological processes.

In response to this criticism, several recent theoretical efforts have appeared that attempt to integrate a range of potential causal variables into the analysis of criminal conduct. Examples include models developed by Elliott, Huizinga, and Ageton (1985); Hawkins, Catalano, and Brewer (1995); Henggeler (1991); Jessor, Jessor, Donovan, and Costa, 1991; Jessor and Jessor, 1977; and Le Blanc, Ouimet, and Tremblay (1988). This approach is also represented in a model we have developed and termed the General Personality and Social Psychological Model of Criminal Conduct (Andrews & Bonta, 1994; Andrews, Bonta, & Hoge, 1990).

3. ☐ A Contemporary Psychological Perspective

The General Personality and Social Psychological Model of Criminal Conduct identifies several levels of variables as causally related to delinquent conduct. The various assumptions and propositions relating to these variables and their

Table 1.2. ☐ Outline of the Major Theories of Criminal Behavior

Neoclassical theories
  Criminal behavior is viewed as willful; individuals engage in criminal behavior because they choose to.

Biological theories
  Criminal acts are viewed as a product of biologically influenced personality, emotional, or behavioral characteristics.

Psychological theories
  Criminal behavior represents deviant behavior that can be explained by means of psychological processes. Psychoanalytic theory and social learning theory are two of the psychological theories particularly relevant to the analysis of criminal behavior.

Economic/sociological theories
  This large group of theories locate the causes of criminal behavior in a social, cultural, or economic context. Marxist, anomie, labeling, and social control theories are prominent examples of this approach.

interaction are developed in detail by Andrews and Bonta (1994) and Andrews et al. (1990), but we will outline the major elements of the model at this point.

At the most immediate level are features of the immediate situation in which the act occurs and is interpreted by the youth. The critical variable here is the perceived balance of rewards and costs associated with the criminal act. The model utilizes social learning theory principles to interpret these dynamics.

At a second level of analysis are four sets of variables that are postulated to impact directly on criminal activity. The first includes variables reflecting the young person's attitudes, values, and beliefs, particularly as they apply to antisocial acts. This has been a relatively neglected type of variable in much criminological research, but it is obviously of crucial importance:

> It is these attitudes, values and beliefs—i.e., procriminal versus anticriminal sentiments—that determine the direction of personally mediated control. They contribute to the standards of conduct that determine whether personally mediated control favors criminal over noncriminal choices. They also represent the pool of justifications and exonerating statements that the person has available in any particular situation. (Andrews & Bonta, 1994, pp. 123–124)

We will note some research supporting the role of attitudinal variables later in this volume.

Antisocial, procriminal associates constitute the second set of immediately causal variables. These associates may include peers of the youth, parents, siblings, or others in the youth's environment. These antisocial associates may impact criminal activity by influencing the youth's reactions to the immediate situation, or they may contribute somewhat more indirectly by fostering the adoption of antisocial attitudes and modes of behaviors.

Behavioral history is included as an immediate causal factor to reflect the importance of the individual's learning experiences. These are of immediate concern because they account for many aspects of the youth's cognitions and behavioral dispositions, and these, in turn, have a direct impact on his or her responses in current situations.

The final set of immediate causal variables identified in the model include aptitude and personality attributes of the youth. Intelligence, psychopathy, impulsivity, neuroticism, and aggressivity are a few of the constructs that have been related to criminal activity. A basic assumption of the model is that a youth's engagement in a criminal act in a particular situation reflects, to some extent at any rate, these more-or-less stable attributes that they bring to the situation.

These four sets of variables constitute, then, the primary causal variables identified in the model. At a third level of analysis are two important factors that operate in a somewhat more distal fashion to affect criminal activity. The first of these includes aspects of the family environment, particularly those relating to parent–child relations. These generally impact criminal activity indirectly through their influence on the youth's attitudinal, personality, and behavioral dispositions.

In other cases, though, the parent may have a more direct impact, as, for example, when lax supervision provides the youth with increased opportunities to engage in criminal acts.

The second of these factors relates to the youth's educational experiences. Academic achievement, school adjustment, and commitment to educational achievement have all been implicated in antisocial activities. The link between these variables and criminal activity is complex, but it is clearly present.

The assessment and treatment implications of the General Personality and Social Psychological Model of Criminal Conduct are best expressed through the four principles of case classification outlined in Table 1.3. The principles are based on the concepts of risk, need, responsivity, and professional override.

Risk factors are those elements of the model that are causally related to criminal activity. Table 1.4 provides a listing of the major risk factors represented in the model and as indicated by the most recent research on the causes of youthful offending. The *risk principle* states that the level of service provided the client should reflect the level of risk that they exhibit. We will show later that the identification of these risk factors constitutes an important challenge in the conduct of psychological assessments.

Need factors are dynamic risk factors amenable to change that, if changed, reduce the risk for criminal activity. Table 1.5 provides a listing of factors that,

---

Table 1.3. ☐ The Risk, Need, Responsivity, and Professional Override Principles

Risk principle of case classification
  Higher levels of service are reserved for higher-risk cases. In brief, intensive service is reserved for higher-risk cases because these cases respond better to intensive service than to less intensive service, while lower-risk cases do as well or better with minimal as opposed to more intensive service.

Need principle of case classification
  Targets of service are matched with the criminogenic needs of offenders. Such needs are case characteristics that, when influenced, are associated with changes in the chances of recidivism. If reduction in the chances of recidivism is an ultimate goal, the more effective services are those that set reduced criminogenic need as the intermediate target of service.

Responsivity principle of case classication
  Styles and modes of service are matched to the learning styles and abilities of offenders. A professional offers a style of service that is matched not only to criminogenic need but also to those attributes and circumstances of cases that render cases likely to profit from that particular type of service.

Professional override
  Having considered risk, need, and responsivity, decisions are made as appropriate under present conditions.

Source: Andrews et al. (1990).

Table 1.4. ☐ **Major Risk/Need Factors within the General Personality and Social Psychological Model of Criminal Conduct**

Antisocial/procriminal attitides, values, beliefs and cognitive–emotional states (i.e., personal cognitive supports for crime)

Procriminal associates and isolation from anticriminal others (i.e., interpersonal supports for crime)

Temperamental and personality factors conducive to criminal activity, including psychopathy, weak socialization, impulsivity, restless aggressive energy, egocentrism, below-average verbal intelligence, a taste for risk, and weak problem-solving/self-regulation skills

History of antisocial behavior evident from a young age, in a variety of settings, and involving a number and variety of different acts

Familial factors that include criminality and a variety of psychological problems in the family of origin and, in particular, low levels of affection, caring, and cohesiveness; poor parental supervision and discipline practices; and outright neglect and abuse

Low levels of personal educational, vocational, or financial achievement and, in particular, unstable employment

Source: Andrews and Bonta (1994).

Table 1.5. ☐ **Promising Targets of Change as Identified in the General Personality and Social Psychological Model of Criminal Conduct**

Changing antisocial attitudes

Changing antisocial feelings

Reducing antisocial peer associations

Promoting familial affection/communication

Promoting familial monitoring and supervision

Promoting child protection (preventing neglect/abuse)

Promoting identification/association with anticriminal role models

Increasing self-control, self-management, and problem-solving skills

Replacing the skills of lying, stealing, and aggression with more prosocial alternatives

Reducing chemical dependencies

Shifting the density of the personal, interpersonal, and other rewards and costs for criminal and noncriminal activities in familial, academic, vocational, recreational, and other behavioral settings so that the noncriminal alternatives are favored

Providing the chronically psychiatrically troubled with low-pressure sheltered living arrangements

Ensuring that the client is able to recognize risky situations and has a concrete and well-rehearsed plan for dealing with those situations

Confronting the personal and circumstantial barriers to service (i.e., client motivation, background stressors with which clients may be preoccupied)

Changing other attributes of clients and their circumstances that, through individualized assessments of risk and need, have been linked reasonably with criminal conduct

Source: Andrews and Bonta (1994).

according the most recent literature, constitute important need factors or promising targets for change. The *need principle* of case classification states that targets of service should be matched with the specific criminogenic needs of the client. We will also demonstrate the importance of assessing these factors later in the volume.

Responsivity factors are those that are not necessarily directly related to criminal activity but that should be taken into account in intervention decisions. Cognitive style, reading ability, psychopathy, anxiety, and motivation for treatment are examples of responsivity factors. As indicated in the *responsivity principle*, these represent important considerations in attempting to select styles and modes of service that will be effective for the individual offender.

In summary, application of the three principles of the General Personality and Social Psychological Model of Crime suggests, first, that decisions about interventions should be based on thorough assessments of the full range of risk, need, and responsivity factors potentially relevant to the youth, and, second, that the interventions should account for responsivity factors and target specific need factors (Andrews & Bonta, 1994; Andrews et al., 1990). The *professional override principle* is included to indicate, however, that final decisions about the client should not be dictated by formal assessment instruments, but, rather, should rest with the individual responsible for the client.

The model we have just described is designed to be both comprehensive and flexible. It is comprehensive in the sense that it includes the full range of variables that have been described in the major theories of delinquency and have emerged as the strongest correlates of delinquent activity in cross-sectional and longitudinal research studies (for reviews, see Andrews & Bonta, 1994; Andrews, Hoge, & Leschied, 1992; Hawkins, Catalano, & Miller, 1992; Henggeler, 1989, 1991; Kazdin, 1987; Loeber & Dishion, 1983; Loeber & Stouthamer-Loeber, 1986, 1987, 1996; Yoshikawa, 1994).

The model is flexible in the sense that it recognizes that the variables affecting criminal activity will vary across individuals and, further, will vary within the individual with their developmental level. For example, associations with antisocial young people may be a critical factor in the criminal activity of one individual but may have no bearing on the activity of another. Similarly, a poor relationship between parent and child may be directly associated with criminal activity in the case of a 12-year-old but may have no direct impact on an older adolescent.

While we feel that this model provides a useful way of conceptualizing the causes of antisocial activity in young people, we recognize certain potential objections. For one, there are other variables implicated in criminal activity to which we have not assigned major significance. These include social class, financial status, ethnic background, family stress, and others. Our argument is that these variables may have an effect on criminal activity in the youth, but that they operate indirectly through the more proximal variables represented in the model.

A second potential limitation relates to a relative neglect of resilience or protective factors within the model. There is some evidence that risk variables confronting the individual may, under some circumstances, be mediated by the presence of protective factors (Hoge, Andrews, & Leschied, 1996; Luthar, 1993; Rutter, 1987, 1990).

A third limitation relates to an acknowledgment that the mechanisms linking various components of the model are not always well understood. For example, it is clear that there is a link between the quality of parent–child relationships and delinquency, but the means by which this operates is not entirely clear. Counter to this is the observation that research and theoretical efforts within social, developmental, and social psychology are proceeding rapidly and that knowledge of child development, particularly relating to antisocial behaviors, is advancing at a rapid pace.

These potential limitations notwithstanding, we feel that the General Personality and Social Psychological Model of Criminal Conduct has important implications for assessment and intervention activities with youthful offenders. These implications are particularly consistent with either the Child Welfare or Modified Justice approach to delinquency. We will explore the implications more fully as we proceed.

Chapter 2

□

Decision Making within Juvenile Justice Systems

We have seen that the treatment of the individual offender within the juvenile justice system may be represented as a series of decisions that occur between the initial police contact through the disposition phase of processing. We have also seen that a number of components are implicit within this decision process:

1. The acceptance of certain goals for the justice system
2. Assumptions about the way in which various alternative courses of action relate to the goals
3. Judgments about the clients and their bearing on these assumptions
4. Final decisions among the alternatives

Three sources of inappropriate or invalid decisions were identified within this framework. These involved incorrect assumptions about alternative courses of action, invalid judgments about the youth, and the inconsistent application of rules within the system. It is the latter two issues that form the primary concern of this volume, and our goal, as we have been, is to show how the use of systematic psychological assessments can be used to enhance the quality of decisions made about the youth by improving the validity of judgments and encouraging the consistent application of decision rules.

Our focus in this chapter is on the decision process as it operates in the juvenile justice system. We begin with an outline of the major types of decisions represented in the system. This is followed by a discussion of the different areas of judgment about the youth and their circumstances that inderlie those decisions. Finally, we discuss the processes involved in forming the decisions and judgments. This then leads to a discussion of the role of psychological assessments in these processes in the following chapter.

1. Areas of Forensic Decision Making

Table 2.1 provides an outline of the major types of formal decisions provided for in juvenile justice systems. While the outline does not have universal appli-

Table 2.1. □ **Major Statutory Decision Areas within Juvenile Justice System**

Police investigation/processing
  Release
  Release with warning
  Arrest
  Arrest/detention
Intake/preadjudicatory processing
  Dismissal
  Release with warning
  Preadjudicatory diversion
  Referral for prosecution
  Detention
Adjudication
  Dismissal
  Waiver or transfer to adult court
  Waiver or transfer to mental health system
  Adjudicatory judgment (guilt/innocence)
Disposition
  Absolute discharge
  Warning/reprimand
  Fine/restitution
  Alternative measure
  Probation
  Open custody
  Secure custody

cability, it is generally applicable to the majority of systems observed in Canada, the United Kingdom, and the United States.

One point we wish to emphasize before we present the overview is that, while much of the decision-making process is guided by statute or administrative guidelines, considerable discretion is often built into the systems. We will return to that point when we discuss decision-making processes later in the chapter.

1.1. Police Investigation/Processing

The initial contact with the youthful offender generally involves the police, although the actual initiation of the action may have begun with a complaint from a parent, the school, a childcare agency, or a member of the public. In any case, and as has often been noted (Doob & Chan, 1982; Frazier & Bishop, 1985; Giller & Tutt, 1987), police are usually provided with considerable discretion regarding the decisions available to them: release, release with warning, arrest (with or without detention). Some jurisdictions also provide for diversion decisions at police discretion.

1.2. Intake/Preadjudicatory Processing

This is the phase following arrest when decisions are to be made regarding further processing of the case. The range of options involved in those decisions are usually specified by statute, with the alternatives generally ranging from absolute dismissal or discharge to referral for prosecution.

There is, of course, considerable variability across juvenile justice systems in the range of alternatives actually available at this level. Thus, some systems provide for a range of preadjudicatory diversion or alternative measures programs, while other confine the choices to discharge or criminal processing. The province of Ontario is an example of a system with a considerable range of alternative measures options: participation in a crime prevention educational program, preparation of an essay or poster, community service activity, apologies to the victim, financial or other compensation to the victim, donations to charity, or participation in a community program.

Another source of variability across systems at this level concerns the involvement of different types of professionals. For example, police and prosecutors bear primary responsibility for intake processing in some jurisdictions, while in other cases nonjudicial childcare professionals such as probation officers might be involved. One feature of the Corporatism Model described in Chapter 1 involves an emphasis on the use of pychologists, social workers, and other nonjudicial professionals at this point in processing.

1.3. Adjudication

Although statutory language varies considerably from jurisdiction to jurisdiction, the broad decision categories available at this phase of the process are relatively limited: dismissal of charges, waiver or transfer to adult court (or mental health system), judgment of guilt or innocence.

Again, however, guidelines regarding these decisions show considerable variability from one legal jurisdiction to another and often present an unclear picture within jurisdictions. For example, statute and case law regarding transfer to adult court or judgments of mental incompetence are often complex and fail to present clear decision-making guidelines. Grisso and Conlin (1984) and Mulvey (1984) have discussed this issue in the United States context, while Bala (1992) and Rogers and Mitchell (1991) have provided discussions relevant to the Canadian setting. We will return to the issue in later chapters.

1.4. Disposition

Table 2.1 presents only in the broadest terms the range of options available for a youth judged guilty of a crime. For example, the range and nature of options available within the alternative measures/community service option varies considerably across jurisdictions. Similarly, there is often considerable variability respecting custody options. In many systems there is a choice between referral to a locked, secure facility or an open custody facility, sometimes with a further range of options within the latter category.

It is important to recognize also that there are other decisions embedded within these disposition categories. These include decisions about the length of sentence mandated for probation or custody, the level of supervision to be provided within the probation option, and the level of security provided in the custody setting. In some cases, the court is also provided with the option of ordering or recommending treatment or counseling within the various alternatives.

The types of alternative dispositions available to the youth court are generally specified by statute. Further, in some cases, more or less specific guidelines are provided regarding the utilization of those dispositions. For example, the principles of the Young Offenders Act of Canada indicates the conditions that should be met before a youth is referred to secure custody. Also, in some jurisdictions specific sentencing guidelines have been introduced. As we will see, however, in most cases considerable latitude exists within systems regarding decision making in these areas.

It is also worth noting that a variety of personnel may be involved in disposition decisions. Final decisions regarding these dispositions are usually reserved for a judge or magistrate, but in many cases other judicial personnel, including prosecutors and perhaps defense attorneys, will be consulted. Also, in many jurisdictions, childcare professionals, including probation officers, social workers, and psychologists, will be consulted on the decision. In fact, in systems requiring a predisposition report, probation officers responsible for preparing the reports may exercise considerable influence on decisions. Finally, systems vary considerably in the assignment of responsibility for supervising the young person while on probation, in treatment, or in custody. Probation officers, social workers, psychologists, childcare workers, and correctional officers may be involved at this level.

2. □ Judgments about the Youth and Their Circumstances

As we have shown, the judicial decisions discussed in the previous section rest in all cases on judgments made about the youth and their circumstances. For example, a policeman's decision to release a child accused of shoplifting may be based on that officer's judgments that (1) the crime was relatively minor; (2) the child seemed remorseful about the crime; (3) a responsible parent appeared when called; and (4) the store personnel were willing to let the officer decide. Similarly, a judge might grant an absolute discharge for a youth accused of a crime on the grounds that (1) it was a first offense and (2) the youth demonstrated a high level of maturity and intelligence. In both cases the decision was guided by a set of judgments made by the judicial officer.

These judgments generally involve inferences about some aspect of the youth's aptitudes, personality, behavior, or attitudes. They may also involve inferences about the crime (e.g., its seriousness), the youth's family situation, or community factors impacting the youth. The judgments may also be discussed in terms of forensically relevant categories.

2.1. □ Seriousness of Offense

Judgments about the seriousness of the criminal act committed by the young person form an important component of the Modified Justice, Justice, and Crime Control models of juvenile justice. Each of these models places more or less emphasis on a sanctioning/punishment component within the juvenile justice system, and each establishes a link between the seriousness of the youth's offense and the processing of the young person. Specifically, the severity of a disposition, including length of sentence, should vary with the severity of the offense. A concern for seriousness of offense also flows from the just deserts form of retribution theory (which underlies, to some extent at any rate, the Justice and Crime Control models). The central principle of the just deserts position is that the nature of the judicial disposition should be directly linked to the severity of the criminal act and the culpability of the offender.

However, while judgments about the seriousness of an offense are important elements within several of the models of juvenile justice, dealing with the construct has proven exceedingly difficult (McDermott, 1983). The major problem is that there is no universally agreed-upon basis for forming the "seriousness" continuum. Even the use of a broad category distinction, such as property vs. person crimes, provides a very problematic basis for judgments of "seriousness." There are many cases in which property crimes may have a greater negative impact than certain violent crimes. To illustrate, the theft of a bicycle from someone completely dependent on that bike by an individual who treated the matter in a cavalier manner would probably be regarded as more serious than an assault on the school grounds involving one student hitting another but immediately expressing regret and remorse for the act.

This example highlights the key aspect of the problem of judging the seriousness of a crime: The significance of a criminal act depends upon a range of factors external to the actual seriousness of the crime, and it is usually acknowledged that evaluations of the act should take account of these factors. We will consider the latter variables as aggravating/mitigating factors in the next section.

Despite these difficulties, both legal and empirical efforts have been made to quantify the seriousness judgments. An example of a legal effort is the Violent Crime Index of the FBI, and the most prominent example of an empirical effort to quantify seriousness may be found in Sellin and Wolfgang's (1964) development of an index that takes into account a variety of factors associated with the impact of the crime (see McDermott, 1983, for a critical discussion of these efforts).

While judgments about seriousness of offenses constitute an important element within the decision process in some juvenile justice processing, it must be said that, to the extent that the focus remains narrowly on the criminal act, the mental health professional probably has relatively little to contribute to the formation of the judgments. Whether the criminal act is regarded as a serious or nonserious one will continue to depend on judicial or philosophical considerations.

2.2. ☐ Aggravating and Mitigating Factors

These terms encompass a broad range of factors that are associated with the criminal act and the person committing the act and that may have a bearing on decisions about the youth at all stages of processing. This type of factor is generally considered to be relevant within all models of criminal justice, with perhaps the exception of those reflecting a Crime Control Model with incapacitation and strong retributive or just deserts orientations.

Aggravating factors are those that magnify the seriousness of the criminal action, while mitigating factors are those that serve to reduce or otherwise ameliorate the perceived seriousness of the offense. Generally speaking, mitigating factors represent the obverse of aggravating factors, and the major general categories of these factors are:

1. Impact on the victim of the crime
2. Degree of violence involved in the crime
3. Prior criminal history of the youth
4. Extent of complicity in the crime
5. Relevant characteristics of the young person (e.g., age, mental status, emotional maturity)

The relevance of judgments about aggravating and mitigating factors to judicial decisions depends in some cases on statutory considerations. Under some circumstances, in other words, laws or policy guidelines specify conditions under which aggravating and mitigating circumstances are to come into play. More often, though, the involvement of these factors at various points in processing are left to the discretion of the judicial officer, and their actual utilization depends largely on the assumptions and values of the professional dealing with the young person. Further, and as we will show later in this chapter, the formation of the judgments usually depends on informal and unsystematic procedures.

We feel that mental health professionals may provide a contribution to the formation of these judgments or inferences in two ways. First, they are often able to use their assessment tools to provide systematic information about specific mitigating and aggravating factors. For example, cognitive disability is sometimes utilized as a mitigating consideration in sentencing decisions, and this is an area in which the psychologist is able to provide valid information. Second, there have been some efforts to develop systematic assessment tools and procedures for quantifying and organizing the aggravating and mitigating factors, and these are potentially useful in ensuring some consistency in assessing this dimension. We will describe these in a later chapter.

2.3. □ Mental Status/Maturity

We are referring to judgments about the presence of mental disorder within the young person and their level of maturity regarding their illegal acts. These judgments are sometimes represented as aggravating/mitigating factors and, as such, are considerations in preadjudicatory and postadjudicatory decisions. There are, however, other ways in which these judgments are involved in judicial decisions. For example, judges in some jurisdictions are able to access treatment orders for mentally disabled offenders. In other cases diagnoses of mental illness or inferences about cognitive and moral maturity are explicitly recognized as considerations in decisions about fitness to stand trial, ability to consent to treatment, and transfers to adult court.

While judgments of mental illness and cognitive maturity sometimes receive explicit acknowledgment in statute, definitions of the constructs are often ambiguous (Rogers & Mitchell, 1991; Webster, Rogers, Cochrane, & Stylianos, 1991; Woolard, Gross, Mulvey, & Reppucci, 1992), and, as we will see later, mental health professionals often have considerable difficulty dealing with the constructs. We will, however, review in a later chapter some developments relevant to their assessment.

2.4. □ Risk Level

Judgments of risk entail the use of information about the young person to predict future behavior. These predictions generally have to do with risk for future criminal activity, violent behavior, or harm-to-self. Risk judgments are involved in almost all stages of the processing of young offenders, but they are particularly relevant to decisions about pre- and postadjudicatory detention. Choices about type of disposition (probation, open custody, secure custody); length of sentence;

and the level of supervision provided within the disposition are often based on judgments about risk levels.

Risk judgments are explicitly recognized in certain of the models of juvenile justice described earlier, particularly the Modified Justice, Justice, and Crime Control models, which exhibit a concern for deterrence. Their role is also recognized in statute or case law in many jurisdictions. For example, there are often more or less explicit guidelines regarding the link between the level of risk or dangerousness exhibited by the young person and the level of custody to be imposed. An illustration is s. 515(10) of the Criminal Code of Canada, which provides the following guidelines regarding the preadjudicatory detention of youth; these state that youths should be referred to custody:

> (a) on the primary ground that ... detention is necessary to ensure ... attendance in court ... and (b) on the secondary ground that ... detention is necessary in the public interest or for the protection or safety of the public, having regard to all the circumstances including any substantial likelihood that the accused will, if he is released from custody, commit a criminal offense or an interference with the administration of justice ...

The guidelines are calling specifically for a risk assessment.

This is an area in which we feel that the mental health professional has a particularly important role to play. Reviews by Baird (1985), Clear (1988), Clements (1996), and Glaser (1987) indicate that in most situations risk judgments are based on unsystematic and intuitive procedures and are of questionable validity. On the other hand, as we will show in a later chapter, considerable advances are being made in the theoretical and empirical analysis of risk and in the development of systematic tools for assessing risk. These developments not only reflect enhanced methodological sophistication, but they also incorporate theoretical and empirical advances being made in analyses of the causes of criminal activity. While most of these efforts are being conducted at the adult level, there are also encouraging developments at the juvenile level, as we will see.

2.5. ☐ Criminogenic Need

The Child Welfare, Corporatist, and Modified Justice models all place considerable emphasis on the goal of rehabilitation. They incorporate, in one form or another, the assumption that a major role of the juvenile justice system is to identify factors within the youth or their situation that are placing them at risk for criminal activity and to attempt to ameliorate those conditions through rehabilitative, therapeutic, or other services. Where this assumption operates, there is a necessity for judgments about the needs of the young person.

This assumption is also recognized in most of the sociological and psychological theories of criminal behavior, although, as we saw earlier, the specific variables identified as causes of criminal activity tend to vary from theory to theory. Thus, the sociological approaches assume in one form or another that the roots of criminal activity rest within the social and economic environment of the young person and that positive changes in this environment will reduce the risk of criminal activity. On the other hand, the psychological theories tend to locate the causes of criminal activity within the individual or the dynamics of their immediate situation.

Because each of these theories focuses on a narrow range of causal factors, they also identify a narrow range of need factors. We saw, however, that a number of more integrative theories of youth crime have appeared and that these incorporate a broader range of factors in their analyses of the causes of youthful criminal activity. We feel that these theories provide a better guide to the identification of criminogenic need factors.

As an example, the General Personality and Social Psychological Model of Criminal Conduct (Andrews & Bonta, 1994; Andrews et al., 1990), which we discussed earlier, attempts to incorporate the full range of causal factors linked to criminal activity that have been identified in the research literature. These are termed risk factors within the model. The model also identifies as need factors a subset of the risk factors. Need factors are dynamic risk factors; that is, they are risk factors that are amenable to change and, if changed, reduce the chances of criminal or other antisocial activity. It is assumed, as we saw, that the effectiveness of interventions with young people depends on a careful matching of treatment choices and criminogenic needs.

We feel that the mental health professional has a particularly important role to play in providing judgments about criminogenic need factors. First, and as we will see in later chapters, there are many established psychological instruments appropriate for assessing both personal attributes (e.g., cognition, personality) and circumstantial factors (e.g., parenting style, family functioning) that have been identified as criminogenic needs. Second, we will also see that there have been a number of recent efforts to develop instruments that help to integrate and synthesize the broad range of need factors that may operate in delinquent youth.

2.6. □ Responsivity and Amenability to Treatment

Responsivity factors refer to characteristics of the youth or his or her situation that, while not necessarily associated with criminal activity directly, are relevant to decisions about the youth. Examples of responsivity factors include intelligence, reading ability, presence of mental illness, and motivation. The assessment of these factors is particularly important in those systems with a rehabilitation focus: Choices among alternative treatments should be guided by information about the youth's responsiveness to different types of intervention.

Where intervention options are clearly specified, and where the factors affecting the youth's response to the options are known, the mental health professional may be said to have an important role to play in assessment activities. The cognitive, personality, and attitudinal dimensions that function as responsivity factors represent areas in which valid and reliable assessment tools are available.

Amenability to treatment may also be considered an aspect of responsivity, and it is a judgment often recognized in statute. The concept refers to the likelihood that the youth will respond to treatment or rehabilitation efforts. The judgment is important because it forms the basis in some jurisdictions for decisions about diversion or transfer to adult court. On the other hand, in many cases statute or case law provide very little guidance regarding the definition of amenability to treatment, and this presents serious problems for mental health professionals attempting to assess the construct (Leschied, Jaffe, Andrews, & Gendreau, 1992; Melton, Petrila, Poythress, & Slobogin, 1987; Mulvey, 1984; Rogers & Mitchell, 1991). However, we will attempt to show in succeeding chapters that there are standardized psychological assessments relevant to inferences about amenability to treatment.

3. ☐ Decision-Making Processes

We have identified in the two preceding sections the various areas of decision making relevant to juvenile justice systems and the types of inferences or judgments about clients that underlie those decisions. We concern ourselves here with the processes whereby judgments are formed about clients and are used as a basis for selecting among the alternative courses of action. Reviews of decision-making processes within justice systems by Binder, Geis, and Bruce (1988); Corrado and Turnbull (1992); Gottfredson and Gottfredson (1988); and Grisso and Conlin (1984) emphasize three conclusions about decision making in this context:

1. Considerable discretion exists with respect to decision activities
2. There is a heavy dependence on informal and unsystematic assessment procedures
3. There exists considerable variability within systems in applications of goals and assumptions

These points have been demonstrated within a wide variety of decision areas, including police processing (e.g., Dannefer & Shutt, 1982; Doob & Chan, 1982); predisposition diversion (e.g., Carrington, Moyer, & Kopelman, 1988; Thomas & Fitch, 1981); and dispositions (e.g., Doob & Beauliea, 1993; Hoge, Andrews, & Leschied, 1995; Niarhos & Routh, 1992; Schissel, 1993).

While decisions within juvenile justice systems are usually guided to some degree by statute and administrative procedures, police, prosecutors, judges, and others are generally permitted considerable latitude in the selection among alternative courses of action. This provision for discretion is, of course, not necessarily undesirable. When dealing with human clients, some provision for flexibility is a necessity. On the other hand, the exercise of discretion encourages the use of inconsistent assessment procedures and variability in the application of decision rules. This, in turn, tends to produce inconsistent decisions about clients and thereby contributes to inequities in the processing of offenders. Since most systems embrace a principle of equitable treatment before the law, this represents an undesirable state of affairs.

The second conclusion from the reviews cited is that within most juvenile justice systems there is a heavy reliance on informal, unsystematic assessments and, in particular, on the use of informal clinical interviews. Unfortunately, there is ample evidence from the psychological literature showing that clinical judgments about human characteristics are often fallible and likely to lead to variable and invalid decisions (Cline, 1985; Dawes, Faust, & Meehl, 1989; Garb, 1989). This has been demonstrated specifically with clinical assessments of mental disorder (Garb, 1989), teachers' assessments of student aptitudes (Hoge & Coladarci, 1989), and personnel officers' judgments of job applicants (Harris, 1989).

While there appear to be no efforts to explore specifically the validity of judgments and inferences formed within the juvenile decision process, there is no reason to believe that these would be any more reliable or valid than those yielded by any other type of clinical assessment. Further, the documented variability in decision making in juvenile justice contexts provides, we feel, indirect evidence of inconsistencies in the process of forming judgments and inferences about offenders.

The issue of the validity of judgments and inferences about the youth is, of course, a serious matter and has a direct bearing on the quality of decisions made about the youth. If, for example, a decision about incarceration depends on an assessment of the youth's risk of reoffending, then the validity of the inference about risk level becomes of critical importance. Similarly, the effectiveness of a decision about providing the youth with a program of therapy depends very directly on the validity of the judgment about the youth's need for treatment. It is our position, then, that the common dependence on unsystematic assessment procedures in juvenile justice systems contributes to invalid inferences about clients, which in turn contributes to inappropriate decisions about youths.

The third conclusion from the reviews cited concerns the inconsistent application of decision rules within systems. This inconsistency arises because personnel within systems often embrace different goals for the system and make different assumptions about the best way of achieving those goals:

> ... juvenile court judges and other decision makers have personal views about appropriate decisions and, therefore, ideology or individual theories are likely to be critically important in explaining why youths are treated so differently, even though the law is the same. (Corrado & Turnbull, 1992, p. 118)

There are numerous empirical demonstrations of this point. For example, Farnsworth, Frazier, and Neuberger (1988) utilized data collected from the following groups of judicial personnel within a state juvenile justice system: intake supervisors, law enforcement officers, state attorneys, judges, social workers, childcare workers, supervisors, and case managers. Representatives of these groups were asked to evaluate a wide range of alternative goals of a juvenile justice system (e.g., protection of society, punishment, rehabilitation). They were also asked to indicate the dimensions they considered most important in forming decisions about youths (e.g., youth's attitudes, parent's attitudes). Their results indicated considerable variability across the personnel types in the ranking of goals and in the identification of factors considered relevant to judicial decision making. Educational background also contributed to variability in responses to these items. Perhaps more interesting, however, is the fact that one can also conclude from the authors' data that variability exists within the professional groups. For example, it is clear that the group of law enforcement officers differed in their identification of preferred goals and their opinions about what characteristics of the youth are relevant to processing.

A second demonstration of the point is provided in a study by Doob and Beaulieu (1993) in which they collected data from a group of youth court judges. The judges were presented with a set of four hypothetical cases involving youthful offenders. After reading the cases the judges were asked to indicate what they would consider an appropriate disposition. They were also asked to respond to a series of questions regarding the importance of various factors in their decision making and to indicate their perceptions of the relative importance of various purposes of sentencing. The results of the study indicated substantial variability among these youth court judges regarding the nature of the disposition considered appropriate for a case, the weighting of various case factors, and the weighting of the alternative goals of sentencing.

Doob and Beaulieu (1993) are careful to point out that some of the variability in judgments can be explained by ambiguities in the Young Offenders Act of Canada, within which these youth court judges were operating. Furthermore, and as we noted earlier, some flexibility (and, hence, variability in decisions) is required in any system dealing with human clients. On the other hand, much of the variability demonstrated in these research studies and in anecdotal reports reflects unacceptable inconsistencies in the application of decision rules and contributes to inappropriate decisions. Also, variability in the application of rules combined with the use of informal assessment procedures provide fertile ground for the operation of bias in the judicial decision-making process and contribute to inequity in the treatment of offenders.

Reviews by Binder et al. (1988), Grisso, Tomkins, and Casey (1988), and Schissel (1993) provide ample demonstrations of the latter point. For example, Schissel (1993) has demonstrated that, contrary to law and policy guidelines, race of youth was, in some cases, a determining factor in both pre- and postadjudicatory decisions within a Canadian youth justice jurisdiction. Inconsistent and inappropriate applications of decision rules were also demonstrated in a study reported by Hoge, Andrews, and Leschied (1995). The results of that study indicated that nonlegal factors relating to family situation and the youth's attitudes had a bearing on referrals to secure custody in a system where the guidelines stated that such referrals were to be based solely on considerations relating to seriousness of offense and risk for reoffending.

In summary, two sources of inappropriate or invalid decisions have been discussed in this section, both arising from provisions for broad discretionary powers. The first relates to the use of informal and unsystematic assessment procedures, and the second to the inconsistent application of decision rules. The central thesis of this volume is that the use of standardized psychological measures and systematic assessment procedures can play an important role in addressing these problems and in improving decision processes within the juvenile justice system. We turn next to a discussion of these points.

Chapter 3 □

The Role of Psychological Assessments in the Juvenile Justice Decision Process

The focus of this volume is on the assessment process as it operates within the juvenile justice system. This process refers to the collection of data about the client and the translation of those data into a judgment or inference. We have also extended the concept of assessment to include the next stage of processing, which involves the use of the inference in selecting among alternative courses of action.

We have seen that the quality of decisions about the youthful offender (and, hence, the effectiveness of the justice system) depends very heavily on the validity of the judgments made about the youth and the care with which that information is used in selecting alternative courses of action. On the other hand, we have also seen that assessment activities in juvenile justice systems are often conducted in an informal and unsystematic manner and, further, that they involve considerable discretion on the part of personnel within the system. This frequently results in a high level of inconsistency in the processing of offenders and in the operation of bias and error, both in the formation of inferences about clients and in the actual decision-making process. The results are inappropriate and invalid decisions about youth.

A basic premise of this volume is that the process of formulating and utilizing assessments within the juvenile justice system can be improved through the use of standardized psychological assessment instruments and procedures. We will discuss these in detail in later chapters but will present at this point an outline of the major types of instruments and procedures with which we are concerned.

1. □ Major Types of Instruments and Procedures

Any measure or procedure used to collect data about an individual and to formulate an inference could be considered a psychological assessment. However, when we talk of standardized psychological assessments we have a somewhat more specific referent. Standardized psychological assessments are those with fixed stimulus, response, and scoring formats and for which psychometric data are available. The Wechsler Adult Intelligence Scale–Revised (Wechsler, 1981), for example, constitutes a structured psychological assessment instrument: Stimulus items, scoring formats, and administration procedures are all standardized, and psychometric data are available for the instrument. A structured interview schedule such as the Hare Psychopathy Checklist (Hare, 1991) is another example of a standardized psychological assessment tool, with its structured set of questions, scoring format, and administration procedures, as well as its supporting psychometric data.

Standardized psychological assessment instruments and procedures show considerable variability in their focus. Areas assessed range from intelligence levels through personality traits to systems for classifying offenders in terms of risk levels. We have organized our discussion of the instruments and procedures in the following chapters into four subject areas:

1. Intelligence, aptitude, and achievement
2. Personality, attitudes, and behaviors
3. Family, community, and therapeutic/correctional environments
4. Diagnostic and classification systems

The instruments also differ in format. Psychological tests or other self-report measures constitute one important class of assessment tools, but, as we will see, rating scales and checklists, interview schedules, and observation schedules are also important. Furthermore, in some cases these instruments are used singly, and in other cases they are combined into batteries. We will also examine some of the more comprehensive diagnostic and classification assessment systems.

It should be understood that there is a continuum of structure in standardized psychological assessments. At one extreme are the actuarial classification systems based on objective data that yield scores derived through mathematical procedures. At the other extreme are semistructured procedures that may call for a higher level of judgment on the part of the assessor; certain of the interview schedules are examples. Still, the line between these structured psychological assessments and the informal, unstructured, intuitive assessment and decision procedures usually observed in the justice system is clear.

Our basic argument, again, is that the process of formulating and utilizing forensic assessments within the juvenile justice system can be improved through the use of standardized psychological assessment procedures. We will develop this argument further in a moment, but first we turn to a discussion of the major bases for evaluating forensic assessments.

2. □ Evaluating Forensic Assessments

The ultimate test of assessments made within the juvenile justice system is whether the evaluation will provide the basis for decisions that, in turn, lead to the achievement of goals embraced by the system. We may ask, for example, whether an assessment leading to a decision to refer a youth to a group home for a period of treatment produced the desired goals of improving the youth's attitudes and school performance and, hence, his or her ability to resist further criminal activity. Unfortunately, this type of criterion is often too remote for our purposes, and, instead, we will discuss the issue of evaluating forensic assessments in terms more directly relevant to our concerns. We begin with a discussion of various sources of professional standards for the use of psychological assessments and follow this with a review of the major terms used in evaluating the measures.

2.1. □ Professional Standards

The *Standards for Educational and Psychological Testing* (American Psychological Association, 1985) constitutes the primary source of standards for the construction, administration, and evaluation of psychological assessments. These guidelines are the product of a collaboration among three professional groups: the American Psychological Association, the American Educational Research Association, and the National Council on Measurement in Education.

The guidelines contained in the *Standards for Educational and Psychological Testing* are phrased in terms relevant to psychological tests, but they actually apply to all psychological measures, including rating instruments, observation schedules, and interview schedules. Four sets of guidelines are included. Part I provides technical standards for test construction and evaluation; included are detailed guidelines relating to validity, reliability, test development, scaling and norming, and publication of manuals and other technical material. Part II provides recommendations regarding test usage. These recommendations cover a very broad range of issues relating to the actual use of psychological measures, including the qualifications of individuals utilizing psychological measures, the need for familiarity with the technical features of the assessments being employed, and the importance of the assessor's sensitivity to unintended consequences of assessments. Part III presents standards for the utilization of assessments with special groups. For example, guidelines are presented regarding the assessment of individuals with reading or other types of language disabilities. Finally, Part IV of the *Standards* provides detailed guidelines regarding the ethical use of psychological assessments, including obtaining informed consent, the release of assessment information, and the use of stigmatizing labels.

While the *Standards for Educational and Psychological Testing* constitute the primary source of standards for the construction, administration, and evaluation of psychological assessments, there are other sources of prescriptions. For example, Division 41 of the American Psychological Association (1991) has formulated a set of recommendations relevant to the conduct of forensic assessments. These guidelines are somewhat less detailed than those just described, but they do provide information about assessment issues arising specifically within forensic contexts.

For example, concrete guidelines are offered with respect to the conduct of risk assessments. Additional guidelines covering the conduct of assessments may be found in the Canadian Psychological Association's *Code of Ethics* (Canadian Psychological Association, 1991) and in *Ethics for Psychologists: A Commentary on the APA Ethics Code* (Canter, Bennett, Jones, & Nagy, 1994).

While the availability of standards regarding psychological assessments is important, the enforcement of the standards is sometimes more problematic. Individuals functioning as professional psychologists generally must be registered with a professional association of psychologists. These operate at the state level in the United States and at the provincial level in Canada. The College of Psychologists of Ontario is an example of such a group. Members of these professional groups are bound by the ethical standards of the group, and these standards generally incorporate the guidelines included in the *Standards for Educational and Psychological Testing* or similar documents. Furthermore, these professional associations have the legal authority to enforce their ethical standards and, in fact, do so when transgressions are brought to their attention. A similar system operates, of course, with psychiatrists and other medical practitioners, although the guidelines regarding assessments would be somewhat less detailed than those of the psychological associations (i.e., see American Psychiatric Association, 1989).

Other professional groupings of psychologists, social workers, and other mental health providers also provide ethical guidelines that would be relevant to the conduct of psychological assessments in juvenile justice settings. However, these organizations often have fewer enforcement powers than legislatively established organizations do. The major problem in this respect, however, is the fact that there are many individuals engaged in conducting psychological assessments who are not members of any professional group of mental health providers and whose activities are completely unregulated. This is recognized as a serious problem in the area.

2.2. □ Evaluation Terminology

The *Standards for Educational and Psychological Testing* and similar guidelines generally depend on the traditional psychometric model for evaluating the assessments, and we will employ that model in our discussions of the various instruments. We might also note that, while the concepts within this model are well known to psychologists and other mental health providers, they may not be well appreciated by other groups of professionals in justice and corrections. Indeed, many mental health providers in justice settings may find that part of their role entails bringing the importance of basic psychometric considerations to the attention of other professionals. This involves what Grisso (1987) refers to as educating the "legal consumer." Key concepts from the psychometric model are identified in Table 3.1. We will provide a brief discussion of each of these concepts here, and the

Table 3.1. □ Definitions of Terms from the Psychometric Model

Term	Definition
Reliability	The stability or consistency of a measure; formally defined as the relative proportion of true and error variance within a measure
Content validity	Adequacy with which a measure represents the conceptual domain it is expected to encompass
Construct validity	Theoretical meaning of scores from a measure; the accuracy with which the measure represents the construct in question
Criterion-related validity	Extent to which scores from a measure relate to a criterion of performance; the two forms of criterion-related validity are concurrent validity and predictive validity
Dynamic predictive validity	The sensitivity of a measure to changes in the dimension being assessed
Incremental predictive validity	Extent to which a measure exhibits improvements in predictions relative to other procedures
Relevance	Extent to which scores from a measure relate to the decision to which they are linked
Utility	The value of improvements in the decision process yielded by the use of a measure relative to the costs of employing the measure

reader is referred to any of a number of standard assessment textbooks for more detailed examinations of the constructs.

Reliability is generally defined in terms of the consistency or stability of a measure. More formally, it refers to the relative proportion of true and error variance within a measure. Reliability is generally evaluated by means of the test–retest, interrater agreement, and internal consistency procedures. Each of these represents a different approach to the analysis of the degree of error present with a measure.

Reliability coefficients are generally expressed through correlation coefficients. These provide indices of the proportion of true and error variance within the measure. A closely related statistic is the standard error of measurement. This index is based on the reliability coefficient, and it provides us with direct information about the degree of confidence with which we can view an individual score from a particular measuring instrument.

It should be emphasized that reliability constitutes an essential consideration in the evaluation of psychological measures. Lack of stability or consistency in a measure seriously interferes with its utility in applied assessment situations.

Validity is a somewhat more difficult construct to define, but in its broadest sense it refers to the meaningfulness of a measure (Messick, 1995). Several different forms of validity have been identified, although there is often some confusion in the literature about the way in which the forms should be defined. As indicated in Table 3.1, we have chosen to deal with five forms of validity.

Content validity refers to the adequacy with which a measure represents the conceptual domain it is expected to encompass. We may ask, for example, how well the items on an intelligence test sample what we consider the domain of intelligence. Similarly, we might attempt to evaluate the adequacy with which an instrument designed to assess risk for violent actions encompasses the range of factors we consider relevant to future risk. Content validity is usually evaluated through subjective procedures, and it is generally not considered a particularly stringent means for establishing validity. On the other hand, this type of evaluation is important in the early stages of developing measures, and it is also sometimes important from the point of view of the clients' acceptance of the legitimacy of a psychological measure.

Construct validity is the second form of validity we have identified, and we note that both Anastasi (1986) and Messick (1989a, 1989b, 1995) have suggested that this form of validity constitutes the key concept in the psychometric model. They have defined construct validity in terms of the theoretical meaning or accuracy of a measure. For example, in the case of an intelligence test, we would raise a question about the actual meaning of the score from the test: Just what does it represent in terms of the cognitive functioning of the individual? The same type of question could be raised of an assessment indicating a diagnosis of Attention-Deficit/Hyperactivity Disorder. The issue in this case would concern the actual implications of that assessment for the functioning and behavior of the individual.

Construct validity is sometimes evaluated in theoretical terms. In this case the operational procedures represented in the measure are evaluated intuitively or inductively with reference to a particular theoretical position. An example would be an evaluation of a test of moral maturity against a theory of moral maturity.

The preferred method for evaluating construct validity in psychology is, however, through empirical means. One statistical procedure used in this case is factor analysis, a procedure capable of providing us with information about the nature of the construct being assessed. For example, factor analyses of behavioral data have been useful in providing valuable information about various dimensions of behavioral pathology. These analyses have shown, for example, that aggression, dependence, social withdrawal, anxiety, and attention problems constitute relatively independent dimensions of behavioral pathology and that these are assessed as independent factors by certain rating scales and checklists. We will look more closely at these measures in Chapter 5.

Other procedures for evaluating construct validity involve relating measures to alternative measures of the same construct. For example, our understanding of the construct of aggression has been advanced through research exploring links among parent and teacher ratings, observational measures, and interview measures of this construct. Similarly, the construct of psychopathology has been clarified through research linking interview, observational, and rating measures of pathology.

The most stringent empirical means for evaluating construct validity involves the multitrait-multimethod procedure, which was originally described by Campbell and Fiske (1959). This method essentially compares the extent to which a measure relates to alternative measures with which it should theoretically be related (convergent validity) with the extent to which it relates to alternative measures with which it should theoretically not be related (divergent validity). For example, if we assume that aggression, anxiety, and attention-deficit disorder are independent dimensions, then a measure of aggression should relate significantly to alternative measures of aggression, but should show no relation (or lesser relations) with measures of anxiety and attention-deficit disorder. This type of procedure is extremely important in the evaluation of measures, but it has also proven valuable in helping us clarify the meaning of our constructs.

It should be emphasized that construct validity is an extremely important concept within psychology, particularly in applied areas such as criminal justice and corrections. We are attempting to measure constructs such as "psychopathology," "risk for violent offending," and "conduct disorder," and we are using our measures of these constructs as a basis for important decisions about individuals. To that extent, it is important that we be able to demonstrate that we have meaningful measures of the constructs.

It is also useful to acknowledge at this point that there is a particular problem in assessing the construct validity of measures employed in forensic assessments. This problem has been discussed by Grisso (1986, 1987); Halleck, Hoge, Miller, Sadoff, and Halleck (1992); Matarazzo (1990); Melton et al. (1987); and Rogers and Mitchell (1991), and it involves the fact that in some cases there is a lack of correspondence between the definition of constructs as derived from psychological theory or research and the definitions represented in the legal system. We will return to this issue later in the volume.

Criterion-related validity is the third form of validity identified in Table 3.1. This is defined as the extent to which scores from a measure relate to some criterion of performance. Two forms of criterion-related validity are concurrent validity (in which predictor and criterion scores are collected at the same time) and predictive validity (in which criterion scores are collected some time after the predictor scores). To illustrate, relating scores from a personality test to information about the current criminal activity of the individual would reflect on the concurrent validity of the personality test, while relating scores on the test to criminal activity assessed 3 years later would reflect on the predictive validity of the personality test.

Predictive validity is of particular concern within forensic assessments because measures are often used as a basis for predicting future behavior. As we will see, for example, numerous efforts have been made to develop risk assessment measures; these are measures that are presumably capable of providing information about the likelihood of future criminal activity.

Evaluations of criterion-related validity are generally based on correlation coefficients and their accompanying confidence indices. For example, the criterion-related validity of a personality test might be expressed as follows: $r = .47, p < .05$. The correlation value of .47 provides us with information about the degree of association between the personality test scores and the criterion of interest, while the confidence index tells us that there are fewer than 5 chances in 100 of obtaining an association of that magnitude under chance circumstances (given a particular number of observations).

There are many cases within forensic assessments, however, where we would like more direct information about the predictive value of scores from our tests or other measures. In these cases contingency tables are often useful. Table 3.2 provides illustrations of the structure of these tables. Part A of the table describes the basic structure of a dichotomous contingency table. Two types of correct decisions are recognized: true positives (positive prediction and positive outcome) and true negatives (negative prediction and negative outcome). There are also two types of misses: false positives (predict positive outcome but obtain negative) and false negatives (predict negative outcome but obtain positive).

Part B of the table presents an example of the use of a contingency table based on hypothetical data. In this case we are forming two predictions of future recidivism for a sample of youthful offenders based on a battery of assessment tools: Scores on that battery place 158 of the 343 youth in the sample in the high-risk group and the remaining 185 in a low-risk group. Recidivism data collected 3 years later then allows us to assess the accuracy of our predictions. The hypotheti-

Table 3.2. □ Illustrations of Prediction Accuracy Contingency Tables

A: Illustration of Terminology

	Actual Outcome	
	Reoffended	No reoffending
Predict reoffending	True positive	false Positive
Predict no reoffending	False negative	true Negative

B: Hypothetical Illustration of a Prediction Accuracy Contingency Table

	Actual Outcome		
	Reoffended	No reoffending	N
Predict reoffending	106	52	158
Predict no reoffending	64	121	185
N	170	173	343

cal data indicate that 170 of the youth were actually charged with new crimes, while an almost equal number (173) present no evidence of new criminal activity.

What we want to know, of course, is the success of our predictions from the assessment tools. Various indices are available for that purpose. For example, we can express the proportion of correct predictions by adding true positives and true negatives and dividing by the total number of predictions. Sixty-six percent of our predictions in the hypothetical case are correct predictions. We can also calculate the percentage of those who recidivated who were correctly identified. The figure was 62% in our sample. As we will see, information of this sort is often considered to be very important in the evaluation of forensic assessments. Other types of indices that may be derived from contingency tables have been presented by Andrews and Bonta (1994); Hart, Webster, and Menzies (1993); and Loeber and Dishion (1983).

Construct and criterion-related validity constitute the major forms of validity, but there are two other forms that have relevance to forensic assessments. Dynamic predictive validity refers to the sensitivity of a measure to changes in the dimension being assessed. This is very important in therapeutic situations where we want to assess changes in the client. Incremental predictive validity is important in the same sense. In this case we are concerned with demonstrating that a measure exhibits an improvement in predictive validity relative to other procedures. An example may be found in efforts to assess the ability of actuarial risk prediction instruments to predict criminal activity relative to the predictions of clinical assessments.

Another construct important to the evaluation of measures used in forensic assessments is that of relevance. Relevance in this context refers to whether or not the information yielded by the measure is relevant to the decision to be made about the young person. This is somewhat separate from the issue of validity, since it is possible for an instrument to be valid but yield information irrelevant to the decision.

Gottfredson and Gottfredson (1988) point out that the answer to the question of relevance depends ultimately on the goals of the decision process and the assumptions made about the best ways of achieving those goals. To illustrate, if the goal of the system is the rehabilitation of young people and it is assumed that improvements in the home environment constitute an important means for achieving that goal, then information about the home environment is relevant to the decision process. If, on the other hand, a just deserts model is guiding the system and it is assumed that the severity of the crime is the only factor that should be considered in making a decision, then information about the home environment would be irrelevant.

Irrelevance of information may be said to affect the decision process in two ways. First, it may simply represent a nuisance or unnecessary expense. Many systems may be considered inefficient because masses of information are collected about clients but are never really used in the decision process. Second, and more seriously, irrelevant information may encourage irrational or inappropriate decisions. The socioeconomic status of the family may have no bearing on the client's criminal activity or on his or her response to different kinds of intervention. On the other hand, the collection of that information in an assessment process may encourage its use within decision making and thereby distort the decision process.

One final basis for evaluating psychological measures should be noted, and this is in terms of utility or cost efficiency. As we will see, the conduct of psychological assessments is sometimes time-consuming and often involves the efforts of professional experts. This sometimes represents a significant monetary cost. On the other hand, it is important to weigh against these costs those associated with the invalid and inappropriate decisions often produced by unsystematic assessments. The monetary and social costs of these decisions is often high as well. We will return to this point later in the chapter.

3. □ Potential Strengths of Standardized Psychological Assessments

We recognize several areas in which standardized psychological assessments may play a positive role in forensic decision making. We note, first, that there is a growing pool of sophisticated tools and procedures available for assessing a wide range of forensically relevant variables, and we feel that the use of these established measures will improve the validity of our assessments and, ultimately, the quality of decisions made within the juvenile justice system. Many of these instruments have been developed within the areas of educational, developmental, clinical, counseling, and organizational psychology, while others have been specifically developed for the criminal justice and corrections fields. We will review these instruments in later chapters and try to demonstrate their relevance to forensic decisions.

Second, we feel that the use of standardized assessments will contribute to consistency in the judicial processing of youths. For example, instead of each probation officer using their own intuitive procedures for assessing a youth's risk for violent offending, the use of a standardized procedure would ensure consistency of assessment across the system and thereby enhance consistency of interventions. This not only helps ensure equity in the treatment of clients, but it may also serve to reduce the operation of bias within the system and, hence, contribute to more rational decision making.

Third, we feel that the use of standardized psychological assessments encourages the specification of constructs represented in assessments, and that this in turn facilitates evaluations of the decision process. To illustrate, all probation offices within a jurisdiction may use assessments of mental competency for preadjudication or disposition decisions, but because each office is using a different intuitive procedure for making the assessment, it is impossible to evaluate the actual basis for decisions. If, on the other hand, all are required to use a particular assessment procedure measuring explicit constructs, a better basis is provided for evaluating the information forming the judgment of mental competency.

A fourth advantage relates to the incorporation of instruments into forensic assessments from other social science areas, and it derives from Grisso's (1987) argument that we should be making more of an effort in the justice field to incorporate substantive advances from other areas of psychology:

> ... research is needed to translate psychological knowledge for forensic application. I am referring here to applied research that will relate principles from basic psychology to legally relevant questions, so that the inferential process in forensic assessments can be more closely tied to the foundations of psychology as a science. (p. 834)

As we will show, the utilization of assessment tools from developmental, educational, personality, and other areas of psychology represent one way of bringing this knowledge to bear on forensic issues.

A fifth advantage of using standardized psychological assessments is that the field provides sophisticated methodological procedures for evaluating the quality of inferences made from the assessment process. Instead of relying on intuitions about the quality of assessments provided by police, probation officers, social workers, judges, and others, we have the tools for evaluating the extent to which they are reliable and valid.

A final argument in favor of the use of standardized psychological assessments relates to the issue of cost-effectiveness. Inappropriate or invalid decisions about clients often represent a poor use of system or agency resources. Keeping a child in custody, providing therapeutic interventions, and providing community supervision are all heavy drains on system resources. The delivery of these services to youths who do not actually need them is a waste of resources. On the other hand, the failure to deliver services where called for may lead to significant social and personal costs. To the extent that standardized psychological assessments lead to improvements in decisions about the youth, more effective uses of system resources will result. We will present some empirical demonstrations of this point in a later chapter.

4. □ Potential Drawbacks of Psychological Assessments

It is also important to acknowledge some limits and potential problems associated with the use of psychological assessments in the juvenile justice system.

We will outline the problems at this point and discuss them further in subsequent chapters.

One problem, although one not inherent within the assessment enterprise, concerns a lack of consensus on the objectives to be embraced within the system and assumptions made about the best way of achieving those objectives. This has a bearing on the issue of assessment because, as Gottfredson and Gottfredson (1988) argue, the information needs of a system are dictated by the objectives of the system:

> It is far easier to conceptualize the information needs of more rational decision making than to achieve them in practice. One reason is the present lack of consensus on objectives at each of the decision points that define the flow of persons through the process. Another is lack of knowledge generally of relative effectiveness of the available alternatives in terms of the objectives chosen, especially as measures of effectiveness may differ for different classifications of persons. (p. 10)

Again, this problem is not inherent within the assessment process, but it does affect the way in which it is applied. Thus, controversies over the selection of assessment tools and procedures often reflect more basic conflicts over the goals of the juvenile justice system.

A second potential problem rests on the argument that a dependence on psychological assessments produces too much of a focus on individual characteristics and too little concern for the broader social environment of the young person. In other words, the psychological instruments can provide us with considerable information about the cognitive abilities of the youth, his or her personality traits, and his or her levels of behavioral and social adjustment, but give us very little information about the family, community, and other ecological factors. This does sometimes represent a limitation with psychological assessments, but we will show in later chapters how recent developments are responding to this point.

A third limitation relates to the possibility that the use of structured psychological assessments will reduce flexibility of decision making within the system. If we recognize that some measure of professional discretion and autonomy is required within a system dealing with humans, there is a danger that an over-rigid assessment format will hinder decision making within the system. This, too, is not a problem inherent within psychological assessments, but it is one that can be dealt with through intelligent applications of assessments.

A fourth objection often heard in connection with the use of psychological assessments concerns the dangers of labeling and "widening the net." As Markwart (1992) points out, this is a particular problem in juvenile justice systems with a mixed rehabilitation and punishment focus. Assessments of treatment needs may identify risk factors that, while not directly related to the criminal activity, may bring forth a more severe response from the system than would normally be the case. Markwart expresses the point as follows in his discussion of predisposition reports providing a broad and detailed assessment of the youth:

> The great emphasis in the report on the personal situation of the young offender ... may also bring to light information which has little relationship to the offense, yet may, because the young person has "problems", encourage a more onerous disposition than would normally be the case for the offense in question. (p. 262)

On the other hand, this is not really a problem inherent in the assessment activity; rather, it is a situation arising in systems without clear goals and procedures.

A fifth potential problem concerns a lack of fit between the constructs measured by psychological assessments and the judgments required within the juvenile justice system (see Grisso, 1986, 1987; Halleck et al., 1992; Matarazzo, 1990; Melton et al., 1987; Rogers & Mitchell, 1991). Most psychological measures are developed in response to needs in educational, organizational, or clinical settings, and the constructs they measure sometimes have only marginal relevance to judicial decision making. For example, waivers to adult court sometimes explicitly require a judgment of the "maturity" of the youth. However, most psychological measures of "maturity" have little real relevance to that construct as defined within criminal statutes. While there is no solution to this problem at present, we will note in later chapters that efforts are being made to address the issue.

Finally, there is a fear on the part of some that an expansion of the use of psychological assessments will be accompanied by an expansion of the role of mental health providers (particularly psychologists) in the judicial system. One's reaction to this possibility depends, in part of course, on one's view of mental health professionals. It also depends, however, on the model of youth justice operating within a system. For example, those systems embracing a just deserts orientation typically assign a small role to mental health providers in the processing of the youthful offender, while advocates of the corporatism model might favour an expansion of their role. In any case, this sometimes represents a point of controversy when the issue of psychological assessments is raised.

We feel that these limitations and potential problems are important, but we also feel that they represent cautions in the use of psychological assessments within the juvenile justice system rather than reasons not to employ the assessments. We will return to some of these issues in later chapters.

5. □ Organization of the Review

The following four chapters discuss various categories of psychological assessment instruments and procedures relevant to the juvenile justice setting. Chapter 4 presents examples of intelligence, aptitude, and achievement tests that have particular relevance to this setting and discusses the general role of this type of instrument in the forensic assessment process. Chapter 5 focuses on instruments designed for assessing personality, attitudes, and behaviors, while Chapter 6 provides a discussion of instruments for assessing aspects of the home and other environments relevant to the youth's functioning. Chapter 6 also includes a discussion of procedures for assessing correctional programs, both community- and institution-based. Chapter 7 focuses on diagnostic and classification systems specifically developed for forensic assessments.

It is important to acknowledge at the outset that we have not attempted a comprehensive review of assessment instruments and procedures. Rather, our purpose is to describe the various types of tools in general terms, discuss their role in forensic decision making, and present examples of instruments and procedures within the various categories. We have endeavored in selecting examples to include the most recent and most advanced techniques and procedures. We have also included in the tables identifying the instruments a source for the measure; in some cases the measures are available from a commercial test publisher, and in other cases a journal reference is provided. A complete list of instruments and procedures discussed in the book may be found in Appendix I, while addresses for the major test publishers are included in Appendix II.

Two other cautions are also in order. We note, first, that many of these tests and procedures are protected by copyright, and they should not be used or reproduced without permission from the author or test publisher. Second, use of some of the instruments requires special training and expertise, and they should not be used by anyone without the necessary qualifications. General guidelines regarding use of the measures by professionals is provided in the *Standards for Educational and Psychological Testing* (American Psychological Association, 1985), while the commercial test publishers are responsible for controlling the distribution of the instruments.

The catalogs of the test publishers are also important sources of information about new instruments and the features of existing instruments. However, for more objective information about the instruments readers are referred to *The 12th Mental Measurements Yearbook* (Conoley & Impara, 1995), Sattler's (1992) *Assessment of Children* (third edition, revised), and *Test Critiques* (Keyser & Sweetland, 1992).

Chapter 4

□

Assessing Aptitudes and Achievement Levels

The first group of instruments we will consider provide for a focus on aptitudes and achievement levels. We consider these as individual assessment instruments at this point, although, as we will show in later chapters, they are often used in conjunction with other instruments in composite classification or diagnostic systems. We begin the chapter with a discussion and illustration of various types of aptitude tests and follow this with a review of measures of academic achievement. The chapter concludes with a consideration of the relevance of these instruments for decision making within juvenile justice systems.

1. □ Aptitude Assessment Measures

While there is some ambiguity in the assessment literature regarding the meaning of the term "aptitude," we will be using it in the very broad sense of referring to underlying abilities or capacities. Our discussion is based on the following categories of instruments:

- Tests of general cognitive ability
- Tests of specific aptitudes
- Neuropsychological assessments
- Vocational aptitude/interest tests

1.1. □ Tests of General Cognitive Ability

Table 4.1 presents examples of three different types of tests of general cognitive ability. Section A of the table identifies a group of individual intelligence tests. All of these instruments are designed to provide a broad and detailed assessment of cognitive functioning in the youth, and all require individual administration by a trained professional.

These instruments are capable of yielding considerable information about a wide range of cognitive capacities in the individual, and they may also be used to identify specific perceptual, cognitive, and academic deficits. In addition, in the

Table 4.1. □ Tests of General Intelligence

A: Individual Intelligence Tests

Test	Source
Detroit Tests of Learning Aptitudes	PRO-ED
Kaufman Assessment Battery for Children	American Guidance Service
Stanford-Binet Intelligence Scale (4th ed.)	Houghton-Mifflin
Wechsler Adult Intelligence Scale–Revised	The Psychological Corporation
Wechsler Intelligence Scale for Children-III	The Psychological Corporation

B: Group Intelligence Tests

Test	Source
Cognitive Abilities Test	Houghton-Mifflin
Henmon-Nelson Test	Houghton-Miflin
Kuhlmann-Anderson Test	Personnel Press
Multidimensional Aptitude Battery	Research Psychologists Press/Sigma
Shipley Institute of Living Scale	Western Psychological Services

C: Performance Intelligence Tests

Test	Source
Goodenough-Harris Drawing Test	The Psychological Corporation
Leiter International Performance Scale	C. H. Stoelting Co.
Peabody Picture Vocabulary Test	American Guidance Service
Raven's Progressive Matrices	Lewis Publishing Co.

hands of a skilled clinician the instruments may yield information about attitudes, motivation level, and personality characteristics.

The Wechsler Intelligence Scale for Children-III (WISC-III) (Wechsler, 1991) serves as an example of this type of instrument. This individual IQ test is appropriate for youths between 6 and 16 years of age. It yields a variety of measures reflecting a wide range of perceptual, cognitive, and academic aptitudes. The basic scores are (1) a full-scale IQ score reflecting overall cognitive functioning; (2) composite scores reflecting verbal and performance cognitive functioning; and (3) a set of scores reflecting specific aspects of functioning, relating, for example, to verbal comprehension, spatial reasoning, and numerical memory. In addition, patterns of subscale scores are used as a basis for identifying various types of cognitive and perceptual disabilities. Poor auditory memory and distractibility are two examples of the latter.

Kaufman (1979) and Sattler (1992) have shown that a considerable literature on this intelligence scale has been built up over the years. The literature is important in two senses. First, it is a source of more-or-less specific guides for the diagnosis of a wide range of sensory, perceptual, and learning problems. As such, WISC-III often constitutes a critical tool in educational and therapeutic decision making. Second, research has made clear that the instrument may be a useful clinical tool. Skilled administrators can utilize observations collected in the assessment setting to form inferences about personality and attitudinal and behavioral characteristics of the youth.

We may also observe that the individual IQ tests identified in Part A of the table are appropriate for use with the full range of mental abilities. This means, for example, that they are capable of identifying youth with exceptional intellectual abilities, sometimes an important issue when dealing with offenders with poor academic records. At the other extreme, the tests are useful in identifying developmentally delayed youth and in estimating the degree of their cognitive delays. We will see in the next chapter that intellectual functioning constitutes only one basis for assessing the competencies of retarded youth, but the instruments do have a role to play in assessing this particular dimension.

All of the individual IQ tests identified in the table are the result of many years of development and refinement. They all demonstrate adequate levels of reliability, and the scoring of the instruments is based on large, representative normative samples. Furthermore, while there is always an issue regarding the meaning of the construct "intelligence," the diagnostic utility of the tests is well established: the instruments do have value from the point of view of diagnosing perceptual, cognitive, and academic deficiencies and predicting academic performance.

There are, on the other hand, three potential limitations associated with these individual IQ tests. First, the tests must be administered on an individual basis, and administration and scoring are time-consuming. Second, they must be administered, scored, and interpreted by a mental health professional with specific training in use of the instruments. Third, questions are sometimes raised about the relevance of the information provided by the tests for forensic decisions. We will return to this point later in the chapter.

Section B of Table 4.1 presents examples of a second type of general cognitive measure, the group IQ tests. These also measure cognitive capacities, but, unlike the individual tests, they can be administered to two or more individuals at a time. In addition, these tests generally require less expertise in administration and interpretation than the individual tests. They are particularly useful, then, in situations where a testing expert is not available.

The Shipley Institute of Living Scale is a very popular example of this type of instrument. This paper-and-pencil test is composed of two sets of items, one based on vocabulary knowledge and the second on reasoning skills. The scale yields scores reflecting those two aspects of cognitive functioning as well as a total IQ score. Administration of the test requires only about 20 minutes, and scoring is quite straightforward.

While these group tests are generally psychometrically sound and more economical to administer than the individual tests, they generally yield less information than the individual IQ tests. Most of these measures provide a single index reflecting the general level of cognitive functioning of the individual relative to their age group. This limits their usefulness as diagnostic devices, although they often have value as screening instruments.

Section C of the table provides examples of nonverbal or performance IQ tests. These are appropriate for administration to physically or language-handicapped individuals who would be unable to cope with the written material presented in the other IQ tests. As such, they are often appropriate in juvenile justice settings where we are sometimes dealing with youths with limited language skills.

The Raven's Progressive Matrices (Raven, Court, & Raven, 1986) is a good example of this type of test. This is essentially a measure of nonverbal reasoning ability that is useful for children and adolescents with language or physical disabilities. Test items all involve the arrangement of figural symbols, and, hence, there is a very limited dependence on verbal instructions or responses. The test yields scores reflecting several dimensions of abstract reasoning ability.

While these nonverbal intelligence tests are important in the assessment of special need youths, in most cases the information they provide about cognitive functioning is limited, and they must be used with an awareness of these limitations. In addition, most of these instruments require individual administration by a professional with special training in use of the measures and with experience in dealing with handicapped youth.

Before concluding this discussion of the general measures of cognitive functioning, note should be made of some important conceptual developments in the field of intelligence testing.

Sternberg's (1985, 1988) Triarchic Theory of Intelligence represents one of these developments. This theory describes mental functioning in terms more comprehensive than those of theories of intelligence previously discussed or as represented on existing intelligence tests. The model is based on three subtheories of cognitive activity. The first is referred to as the contextual subtheory, and it reflects the assumption that definitions and assessments of intelligence must be based on the extent to which the individual is adapting to the demands of their own environment. The second component is labeled the componential subtheory, and this incorporates a description of the actual processes involved in mental functioning. Finally, the experiential subtheory reflects the assumption that a true test of intelligence should be based on the individual's ability to confront and solve novel problems.

The second important theoretical development is represented in Gardner's (1983) Theory of Multiple Intelligences. This theory also seeks to expand the conceptual range of the concept of intelligence, but Gardner's approach is somewhat different than that of Sternberg. Gardner postulates the existence of seven distinct intelligences: linguistic, logico-mathematical, spatial, musical, bodily-kinesthetic, intrapersonal, and interpersonal. The latter two forms of intelligence reflect the ability of individuals to objectively analyze the feelings, motivations,

Table 4.2. □ Specialized Aptitude Tests

Test	Source
Classroom Reading Inventory	Wm. C. Brown
Illinois Test of Psycholinguistic Abilities	University of Illinois Press
Keymath Diagnostic Arithmetic Test	American Guidance Service
Test of Auditory Comprehension of Language	DLM Teaching Resources
Woodcock–Johnson Psycho-Educational Battery	DLM Teaching Resources

attitudes, and behaviors of themselves and those in their environment. It is important to note that only the first three of these forms of intelligence are normally represented in the available standardized intelligence tests.

Neither of these theories have been translated into practical assessment instruments, and, as should be obvious, there are serious practical problems in doing so. However, they do represent important developments in the sense of offering definitions of intelligence broader than those represented in our available tests, with their focus on academically relevant cognitive processes. They might be viewed as particularly relevant when assessing youthful offenders if the concern is with the ability (or inability) of the youth to perceive and analyze personal and interpersonal problems in positive ways. In any case, practitioners are advised to track developments in this area.

1.2. □ Measures of Specific Aptitudes

Table 4.2 presents examples of another type of aptitude measure, those directed toward the assessment of specific aptitude areas. The focus in some of these tests is on perceptual and performance deficits involving visual, auditory, or speech activities; in others the concern is with the identification of disabilities associated with specific areas of academic performance, particularly reading and arithmetic.

The Test of Auditory Comprehension of Language–Revised (Carrow-Woolfolk, 1985) is an example of an aptitude test designed to measure a specific area of functioning, the ability to comprehend spoken language. The test involves presenting the youth with a stimulus word or sentence to which he or she responds by selecting from among an array of pictures. It assesses the youth's ability to comprehend words and increasingly complex phrases.

The Classroom Reading Inventory (Silvaroli, 1986) is an example of a test designed to measure a specific academic aptitude. This individually administered aptitude test provides information about the current reading level of the youth relative to his or her age and also provides information about specific reading problems. An interesting feature of the measure is that it provides a means for placing the child into educationally meaningful categories. Three categories are included:

1. Independent level showing the grade level at which the youth reads accurately and comfortably
2. Instructional level at which the youth reads and comprehends accurately with teacher guidance
3. Frustration level, which is the grade level at which accuracy drops below criterion

The test also provides for an assessment of listening capacity.

One limitation associated with these specialized aptitude tests is that they generally must be administered by an individual with special training. Also, as Sattler (1992) notes, only limited reliability and validity data are available for many of these measures. However, when used with care, these instruments are capable of yielding valuable information about the cognitive capacities of the youth.

1.3. ☐ Neuropsychological Assessments

There are occasions in dealing with young offenders where some form of brain damage or dysfunction is suspected and considered to be a contributing factor in their poor judgment or inappropriate behavior. The diagnosis of subtle brain dysfunction is often based on an extensive neuropsychological assessment. This evaluation typically investigates the sensorimotor, perceptual, language, memory, and cognitive abilities of the person to determine their adaptive capacity. Sattler (1994) has described the role of neuropsychological assessments in this diagnostic process as follows:

> A wide spectrum of psychological deficits, varying in nature and degree, accompany brain injury in children. Although a neuropsychological assessment may not establish the specific nature, site, and extent of an underlying brain lesion, it can accurately determine the sensory, motor, and mental deficits that may be present. Neuropsychological assessment batteries provide information about verbal and nonverbal intellectual abilities and perceptual-motor abilities, including vocabulary, comprehension, concept formation, memory, perception, and motor skills. (p. 695)

We don't intend to treat these tests in detail but will provide some general observations.

The Halstead-Reitan Neuropsychological Test Battery for Older Children (Reitan & Wolfson, 1985) is an example of a comprehensive neuropsychological assessment battery. This widely used battery is composed of items adapted for children and adolescents from the adult version of the Halstead Neuropsychological Test Battery and has been extensively used with young people with learning problems, head injuries, and a variety of neurological disorders. Academic achievement tests and the WISC-III (Weschler, 1991) are also usually administered with the battery.

Other neuropsychological assessment batteries are less comprehensive than the Halstead but are still capable of serving as screening instruments in the identification of neurological dysfunction. An example is the Quick Neurological Screening Test, which is a brief, individually administered screening test for assessing 15 areas of neurological functioning. The latter include maturity of motor development, spatial organization, and auditory perception. The measure also provides an index of attentional capacity.

Sbordone (1991) has described the forensic use of neurological tests, while critical reviews of the instrument are available from Kolb and Whishaw (1985), Lezak (1995), Sattler (1992), and Valcuikas (1995). Two important points are highlighted in their discussions. First, there remain some questions regarding the reliability and validity of these assessment tools. To this extent they must be used with some caution, particularly when employed in the diagnosis of brain injury. Second, the administration and interpretation of the scales is complex and generally require high levels of training and experience. The batteries should be administered by specialists in neuropsychological assessments. Registration with the American Board of Clinical Neuropsychology is also required in the United States.

1.4. □ Vocational Aptitude and Interest Tests

Another group of instruments are specifically designed for collecting information relevant to educational and career decisions and, hence, are important components of counseling activities. There are actually two types of measures represented in this group; the first includes measures of vocational interests and values, while the second includes measures assessing aptitudes and competencies relevant to educational and vocational pursuits. Table 4.3 presents examples of both types of instrument.

The Jackson Vocational Interest Survey (Jackson, 1994) is an example of an instrument designed to match the interests and values of the young person with different occupations. The paper-and-pencil test consists of 289 pairs of statements describing job-related activities. Respondents indicate a preference between the two choices. Scores from the measure provide detailed information about the way in which the youth's current interests match a wide variety of occupational and educational pursuits.

The second type of measure within this category attempts to assess the extent to which the individual possesses the aptitudes for success in educational and occupational pursuits. The aptitude measures already reviewed in this chapter have important roles to play in such assessments, but there are also some instruments specifically designed to provide information relevant to these choices.

Table 4.3. ☐ Tests of Vocational Aptitudes and Interests

Test	Source
Armed Services Vocational Aptitude Battery	United States Department of Defense
Bennett Mechanical Comprehension Test	The Psychological Corporation
Career Assessment Inventory	Interpretive Scoring Systems
Differential Aptitude Test	The Psychological Corporation
Jackson Vocational Interest Survey	Research Psychologists Press/Sigma
Occupational Aptitude Survey and Interest Schedule	PRO-ED
Self-Directed Search Inventory	Psychological Assessment Resources
Strong-Campbell Interest Inventory	Consulting Psychologists Press

There are a large number of these aptitude tests available. Some, such as the Bennett Mechanical Comprehension Test, are designed for specific occupations, while others have more general relevance. An example of the latter is the Armed Services Vocational Aptitude Battery published by the United States Department of Defense. This instrument was originally developed for selection and placement of armed services personnel, but it is also used widely in educational and career counseling of adolescents. The instrument consists of ten subtests: general science, arithmetic reasoning, word knowledge, paragraph comprehension, numerical operations, coding speed, auto and shop information, mathematics knowledge, mechanical comprehension, and electronics knowledge. Various scores are obtained. These include, first, three composite scores reflecting verbal, mathematical, and academic ability. Second, composite scores reflecting four occupational groupings are derived: mechanical and crafts, business and clerical, electronics and electrical, and health and social. Finally, a composite measure reflecting general ability is derived.

2. ☐ Measures of Academic Achievement

Achievement tests are designed to assess the extent to which the individual has acquired a body of knowledge or set of skills. We might want to assess, for example, the degree to which a youth has mastered the mathematical procedures taught at the sixth-grade level or the level of skill he or she exhibits following a course in computer usage.

Table 4.4 provides a list of widely used standardized achievement tests. The Kaufman Test of Educational Achievement (Kaufman & Kaufman, 1985) is a good example of an individually administered test appropriate for youths between ages 6 and 18. The test provides scores for the following achievement areas: reading decoding, reading comprehension, mathematics applications, mathematics com-

Table 4.4. □ Tests of Academic Achievement

Test	Source
Kaufman Test of Educational Achievement	American Guidance Service
Peabody Individual Achievement Test–Revised	American Guidance Service
Stanford Achievement Test	The Psychological Corporation
Wide Range of Achievement Test–Revised	The Psychological Corporation

putation, and spelling. Both age and grade equivalent scores are provided to aid in interpretation.

While the majority of these standardized achievement tests are well developed and display satisfactory reliability and validity levels, there is a caution with respect to their use. The normative data on which their scoring is based reflects a particular population of individuals, and those data may not necessarily be relevant to the population from which the youth is drawn.

3. □ The Role of Aptitude and Achievement Measures in Juvenile Justice Systems

There are several areas of forensic decision making in which these aptitude and achievement measures are relevant. First, information about mental or cognitive competence is often a consideration in mitigating judgments and, as such, is involved in a variety of pre- and postadjudicatory decisions. For example, diminished mental capacity is often an informal consideration in decisions of whether or not to lay a charge against the youth or to grant an absolute discharge. Judgments about cognitive functioning may also be involved in preadjudicatory and adjudicatory decisions about competency to stand trial or to consent to treatment, and here the judgments may constitute formal components of the judicial process. Similarly, decisions about waivers to adult court nearly always require judgments about mental status or competency. This is illustrated in the Canadian Young Offenders Act, which requires an assessment of mental functioning as part of any decision regarding transfer to an adult court.

Information from both individual and group intelligence tests and certain other types of specialized aptitude tests are relevant to the judgments of mental status or maturity that underlie these decisions. At a minimum, these tests provide objective information about the general reasoning abilities of the youth. Also, because the tests are primarily norm-referenced, they provide information about the cognitive functioning of the youth relative to other age groups. It is possible, for example, to indicate that a 12-year-old's reasoning and memory abilities are comparable to that of the average 6-year-old.

Furthermore, and as we have seen, the individual IQ tests and certain of the specialized aptitude tests are capable of providing more specific information about cognitive functioning, and this too may be useful in forming forensically relevant mental status judgments. For example, the tests can be used to provide accurate assessments of reading ability, and this might be a consideration regarding competency to stand trial. Attention-deficit disorder, learning disability, brain injury, and language deficits may also be assessed with these instruments, and these too are often relevant to decisions requiring judgments about mental competence or cognitive maturity.

Information from both aptitude and achievement tests may also be relevant to judgments about risk levels. This is important because, as we have seen, risk for continued criminal activity often constitutes an important consideration in both pre- and postadjudicatory decisions. Both low intelligence and academic failure have been linked to delinquent activity (Crealock, 1991; Hirschi & Hindelang, 1977), and the careful assessment of cognitive and academic functioning with standardized aptitude and achievement tests should be central to any risk evaluation.

We have also seen that judgments about criminogenic need factors constitute important considerations in decision making within many juvenile justice systems, particularly those with a child welfare and rehabilitation focus. Deficits in cognitive functioning, academic and vocational aptitudes, and academic performance are often recognized as important need factors in the case of the youthful offender. As we saw in Chapter 1, these have been closely linked with criminal activity, and, hence, any efforts to develop realistic intervention plans should be based on careful assessments in these need areas. The tests described in this chapter have important roles to play in these assessments.

We have also argued that intervention decisions should take account of amenability to treatment and responsivity considerations. The General Personality and Social Psychological Model of Criminal Conduct (Andrews & Bonta, 1994; Andrews et al., 1990) discussed earlier emphasizes the importance of considering the youth's cognitive abilities in intervention and treatment decisions. Information from standardized aptitude, vocational, and achievement tests are often of critical importance in selecting among alternative strategies. In a later chapter we will review some models specifically linking cognitive functioning with specific interventions. Similarly, decisions about amenability to treatment require assessments of cognitive, academic, and other skills.

We conclude this chapter by emphasizing three cautions that have already been noted in connection with these aptitude and achievement measures. First, while all of the measures reviewed in this chapter represent more-or-less lengthy periods of development and evaluation, there are still limits associated with their psychometric properties. These limits by no means negate the use of the measures, but they do indicate that they be used with awareness of the limitations.

The second caution is related, and it is to the effect that many of these aptitude and achievement measures require considerable training in administration and interpretation. This requirement varies with the different types of instruments, but aptitude assessments generally represent a rather specialized activity.

Our third caution concerns the use of scores from the aptitude measures in forming forensic judgments or inferences. As has been discussed by Grisso (1986), Halleck et al. (1992), Melton et al. (1987), and Rogers and Mitchell (1991), there is sometimes a discrepancy between the constructs being assessed through these instruments and the legal constructs in question. For example, the construct of cognitive competence as assessed through an intelligence test may not correspond exactly to the construct of competency to stand trial as specified in statute. Similarly, statutes and policies relating to decisions to transfer youth cases to adult court often contain, as we have seen, provisions relating to cognitive maturity. However, the legal definition of cognitive maturity usually has a much more specific referent than that represented in the psychological aptitude tests. We return to this point in a later chapter.

Chapter 5   □

Assessing Personality, Attitudes, and Behaviors

We will consider in this chapter a group of instruments designed to assess aspects of the youth's personality, behavior patterns, and attitudes. The personality measures provide information about relatively stable dispositions of the individual; depression, psychosis, and psychopathy are representative of the constructs encountered in these measures. A second set of measures are based on rating scale and checklist formats. These are designed for the collection of information on overt behaviors and attempt to characterize the youth in terms of constructs such as conduct disorder, social withdrawal, or anxiety. The third set of measures include structured and semistructured interview schedules for assessing personality traits and behavioral dispositions, while a fourth set, the attitudinal measures, attempt to assess cognitions that the young person holds regarding issues such as criminal activity, the courts, and drug use.

We stress again that our selection of instruments in the various categories is not designed to be comprehensive. However, we have attempted to select examples that are the object of current research activity and that have been shown to have some relevance to the juvenile justice setting. Further discussions of these measures may be found in Mash and Terdal (1988), Meyer and Deitsch (1996), Sattler (1992), and the *Test Critiques* and *Mental Measurements Yearbook* series cited earlier. It should also be noted that the instruments are considered as individual measuring tools in this chapter, although, as we will see later chapters, they are often used as components of larger assessment batteries or diagnostic systems.

1. □ Personality Tests

This category includes self-report types of measures designed to assess stable personality traits of the youth. Most of these are in the form of paper-and-pencil tests, although an increasing number are being adapted for computer administration and scoring. Some of the instruments require a fairly high level of technical expertise for administration, scoring, and interpretation.

Table 5.1 identifies six standardized personality tests that have relevance to

Table 5.1. ☐ Personality Tests

Measure	Source/reference
Basic Personality Inventory	Research Psychologists Press/Sigma
High School Personality Questionnaire	The Psychological Corporation
Jesness Inventory	Consulting Psychologists Press
Millon Adolescent Personality Inventory	National Computer Systems
Minnesota Multiphasic Personality Inventory–Adolescent	National Computer Systems
Personality Inventory for Youth	Western Psychological Services
Reynolds Adolescent Depression Scale	Psychological Assessment Resources

the assessment of juvenile offenders. Two of those instruments, the Jesness Inventory and the earlier version of the Minnesota Multiphasic Inventory–Adolescent (MMPI-A), form the basis for more comprehensive classification systems and are discussed later in Chapter 7.

The Basic Personality Inventory (BPI) (Jackson, 1995) may serve as an example of this type of instrument. This 240-item personality inventory is appropriate for administration to youths with at least a grade 5 reading competency. Scoring is based on 12 scales: hypochondriasis, depression, denial, interpersonal problems, alienation, persecutory ideas, anxiety, thinking disorder, impulse expression, social introversion, and self-depreciation.

Jackson (1995) has also derived seven profile types on the basis of data collected from samples of young offenders. These are termed mental health maladjustment, interpersonal maladjustment, antisocial delinquency, somatic complaints, high-risk rebelliousness, defensive denial, and random responding. The latter two function as validity scales in the case of this measure. These profile types are represented as distinct patterns on the 12 basic scales. Considerable support for the psychometric soundness of this instrument has been presented (Jackson, 1995), while Jaffe, Leschied, Sas, and Austin (1985) and Leschied, Austin, and Jaffe (1988) have demonstrated that scores from the instrument have utility in assessments of young offenders.

Most of the tests listed in Table 5.1 yield scores reflecting dimensions of personality similar to those assessed in the BPI. Some yield additional information. For example, the Millon Adolescent Personality Inventory (MAPI) (Millon, Green, & Meagher, 1982) yields several types of scores, including those reflecting (1) the youth's personality style, (2) areas of concern on the part of the youth, and (3) aspects of behavioral adjustment. Definitions of scores within those categories are presented in Table 5.2. The extensive literature associated with this measure provides considerable guidance for its use with clinical samples of young people (Woodward, Goncalves, & Millon, 1994).

Table 5.2. □ **Millon Adolescent Personality Inventory Scale Descriptions**

	Descriptive characteristics
Personality styles	
Introversive	Quiet and unemotional; interpersonally remote due to indifference toward others
Inhibited	Shy; socially ill at ease; lonely, yet keeps to self due to fear of rejection
Cooperative	Avoids asserting self; letting others take the lead; plays down own achievements and underestimates own abilities; kind and sentimental in relationships
Sociable	Talkative; charming; dramatic and emotionally expressive; easily bored with routine and long-term relationships
Confident	Rarely doubtful of own self-worth; seen by others as self-centered and egocentric; takes others for granted
Forceful	Tends to lead and dominate; strong-willed and tough-minded; blunt, unkind, and impatient with others
Respectful	Rule-conscious, serious-minded, and efficient; lives orderly life; avoids unexpected and unpredictable situations; behaves properly
Sensitive	Unpredictable shifts of mood; negative attitude; discontented
Expressed concerns	
Self-concept	Clarity of one's identify or self-image
Personal esteem	Level of satisfaction with oneself
Sexual acceptance	Attitudes regarding emerging sexuality and its associated impulses
Peer security	Feelings of acceptance by one's peers
Social tolerance	Degree of empathy of others, especially peers
Family rapport	Degree of conflict and tension with family members
Academic confidence	Extent to which one feels comfortable and/or satisfied with school performance
Behavioral correlates	
Impulse control	Degree of control over problematic impulses
Societal conformity	Inability or unwillingness to comply with social regulations
Scholastic achievement	Influences resulting in underachievement
Attendance consistency	Signs of either school phobia or school truancy

Source: T. Millon, C. J. Green, and R. B. Meagher, Jr., (1982). *Millon Adolescent Personality Inventory Manual*. Minneapolis, MN: National Computer Systems. Used by permission of National Computer Systems.

All of the tests included in Table 5.1 are well-established instruments with adequate norms (including, in some cases, norms for delinquent groups) and considerable information regarding psychometric properties. In general, the instruments exhibit satisfactory levels of reliability. Validity support, on the other hand, is sometimes more problematic. While most of the instruments present evidence regarding construct and criterion-related validity, questions sometimes remain regarding the actual meaning of the personality and behavioral constructs yielded by the instruments. Also, the dynamic validity of the measures has not always been well established, and this limits their utility for tracking changes in the client over time. The instruments should be used, then, with a full understanding of their limits.

Table 5.3 provides examples of another type of personality measure, which provides for the assessment of self-concept. Self-concept refers, in very general terms, to the individual's self-image. A somewhat more specific definition refers to "... our attitudes, feelings and knowledge about our abilities, skills, appearance, and social acceptability" (Byrne, 1984, p. 429). Self-esteem represents one dimension of self-concept, and it refers more specifically to the way in which the individual evaluates his or her image. The issue of self-esteem is often important in counseling young offenders, as we are often dealing with youth who are suffering from either inflated self-esteem or a poor self-concept.

As Byrne (1984, 1996) and Hoge and Renzulli (1993) have shown, there is considerable controversy over the definition of self-concept. These debates revolve around the way in which different components of self-concept should be defined and the meaningfulness of a global self-esteem construct. These controversies aside, the various measures identified in Table 5.3 can provide useful information about the way in which youths view their attributes and the level of self-esteem they feel toward themselves.

The Multidimensional Self-Concept Scale (Rotatori, 1994) is representative of this type of instrument. This 150-item self-report measure assesses six dimensions of self-concept: social skills, competence, feelings, academic performance, physical appearance, and family functioning. This instrument was specifically developed as a clinical tool, and considerable data are presented in its manual, which supports its reliability and validity. Other instruments assess a broader range of self-concept areas. For example, Marsh's (Marsh & O'Neill, 1994) Self-Description Questionnaire assesses three areas of academic self-concept (reading, mathematics, and general school performance) and four nonacademic areas (physical ability, physical appearance, peer relations, and parent relations). This, too, is a well-researched measure. A detailed review of these and other self-concept instruments is provided by Byrne (1996).

Table 5.3. □ Measures of Self-Concept

Measure	Source/reference
Cutlure-Free Self-Esteem Inventory	Research Psychologists Press
Multidimensional Self-Concept Scale	PRO-ED
Piers-Harris Children's Self-Concept Scale	Western Psychological Services
Self-Description Questionnaire	Marsh and O'Neill (1984)
Self-Esteem Index	Psychological Assessment Resources

2. □ Behavioral Ratings and Checklists

Another type of instrument is based on a rating scale or checklist format and is designed for assessing dimensions of social, emotional, or behavioral competence. These measures are generally based on reports of overt behavior provided by the youth (self-report measures) or by an individual acquainted with the youth (parent, teacher, peer, childcare worker, clinician). We have divided these into three subcategories for purposes of discussion. The first includes those directed toward the assessment of social or behavioral pathologies. A second category of instruments are all self-report measures focusing specifically on criminal and other deviant or self-destructive activities. The third category includes adaptive behavior measures designed specifically for assessing developmentally delayed youth.

2.1. □ Measures of Social and Emotional Competence and Pathology

Table 5.4 presents examples of behavioral instruments designed for assessing dimensions of social, emotional, and behavioral competence and pathology. The Revised Behavior Problem Checklist (RBPC) (Quay & Peterson, 1987) is an example of this type of instrument. This 85-item checklist is designed for completion by a knowledgeable observer (parent, teacher, childcare worker, clinician). Items refer to relatively specific overt behaviors (e.g., "disruptive; tendency to annoy and bother others"; "temper tantrums"). The scale yields a total score reflecting the youth's overall level of behavioral maladjustment as well as six factor scores: conduct disorder, socialized aggression, attention problems–immaturity, anxiety–withdrawal, psychotic behavior, and motor tension excess.

Table 5.4. □ Behavioral Measures of Social and Emotional Competence

Measure	Source/reference
Adjustment Scale for Children and Adolescents	McDermott, Marston, and Stott (1993)
Behavior Assessment System for Children	Reynolds and Kamphaus (1992)
Brief Psychiatric Rating Scale for Children	Overall and Pfefferbaum (1982)
Child Behavior Checklist (Parent)	University Associates in Psychiatry/Guidance Centre
Child Behavior Checklist–Teacher Report Form	University Associates in Psychiatry/Guidance Centre
Conners Teacher Rating Scale	Multihealth System
Devereux Adolescent Behavior Rating Scale	Devereux Foundation
Revised Behavior Problem Checklist	Quay and Peterson (1987)
Youth Self-Report Inventory	University Associates in Psychiatry/Guidance Centre

The manual for the instrument includes normative data from several clinical and nonclinical groups to aid in scoring. We might also note that the earlier version of this instrument, the Behavior Problem Checklist, forms the basis for a correctional classification system; this will be discussed in Chapter 7.

The Child Behavior Checklist (Achenbach, 1991a) and Child Behavior Checklist-Teacher Report Form (Achenbach, 1991b) yield factor scores similar to the RBPC, but these instruments are particularly interesting because they are part of a family of parallel instruments. These include the parent, teacher, and self-report versions (Youth Self-Report Inventory) identified in the table. Also included are a standardized observation schedule (Direct Observation Form) (Achenbach, 1991b) and an interview schedule (Semistructured Clinical Interview for Children) (McConaughy & Achenbach, 1990). The availability of these parallel forms permit the collection of information about the emotional and behavioral adjustment of the youth through a variety of formats and sources. A similar concept is represented in the Behavior Assessment System for Children (Reynolds & Kamphaus, 1992). This multidimensional/multimethod system is designed for assessing behavioral competency in children and adolescents. It is composed of behavioral rating scales designed for completion by teachers, parents, and the youth as well as an observation schedule and a developmental history interview.

All of the instruments listed in Table 5.4 are the object of current research activity, and considerable evidence is available regarding their psychometric properties. All display adequate levels of reliability and criterion-related validity, and normative scores from clinical and nonclinical groups are available to aid interpretation. However, as with all measures of personality and emotional competence and pathology, questions sometimes remain about the validity of the instruments. For example, questions have been raised about the meaningfulness of the conduct disorder construct yielded by some of these instruments (Hoge & Andrews, 1992; Waldman, Lilienfield, & Lahey, 1995). An awareness of this caution is particularly important when using the instruments for labeling and placement purposes.

2.2. ☐ Measures of Antisocial and Self-Destructive Behaviors

Table 5.5 provides examples of another type of behavioral measure. These are self-report checklists or rating scales designed to provide information about antisocial activities or self-destructive behaviors. Several of these measures are designed to provide information about delinquent activities. An example is Mak's (1993) Self-Reported Delinquency Scale. The scale solicits information from the youth regarding the extent to which they have engaged in a wide range of minor and serious criminal activities. While measures of this type based on self-disclosed information must be viewed with some caution, there are circumstances under

**Table 5.5. □ Self-Report Measures of Delinquent and
Self-Destructive Behaviors**

Measure	Source/reference
Adolescent Drinking Index	Research Psychologists Press/Sigma
Antisocial Behaviours Scale	Forth and Brown (1993)
Drug Abuse Screening Test	Skinner (1982)
Drug Use Screening Inventory	Tarter (1990)
Eating Disorder Inventory–2	Garner (1996)
Self-Report Delinquency Scale	Elliott et al. (1989)
Self-Reported Delinquency Scale	Mak (1993)
Suicidal Ideation Questionnaire	Research Psychologists Press/Sigma

which they can provide useful information about the youth's criminal activities (Elliott, Huizinga, & Menard, 1989). Other instruments included in the table are designed to provide information about specific problem behaviors, including drug and alcohol abuse, risk for suicide, and eating disorders.

2.3. □ Measures of Adaptive Functioning

There are occasions in dealing with young offenders when mental retardation is suspected or confirmed and an assessment of the competence of the youth is needed. This need may arise in connection with judicial decisions or in association with counseling or therapeutic decisions. The aptitude measures reviewed in the previous chapter have, of course, an important role to play in assessing developmentally delayed youth. However, efforts have also been made to develop measures for providing a broader assessment of the behavioral competencies of the individual. Table 5.6 provides examples of this type of tool. Most of the instruments are based on rating or checklist format and are designed for completion by teachers, clinicians, or childcare workers knowledgeable about the child.

The Vineland Adaptive Behavior Scales (Sparrow, Balla, & Cicchetti, 1984) is an example of this type of measure. The instrument is designed for assessing the competence of developmentally delayed and other handicapped individuals. It is in the form of a questionnaire designed for completion by an individual familiar with the youth, although it may be administered in an interview format as well. The scales are designed to assess adaptive skills in four areas: communication, daily living activities, social interactions, and motor activity.

All of the instruments identified in Table 5.6 are the result of many years of development and evaluation, and all are capable of providing useful information about the functioning of cognitively handicapped youth. On the other hand, discussions of these measures by Hallahan and Kaufman (1991) and Sattler (1992)

Table 5.6. □ Measures of Adaptive Functioning

Measure	Source/reference
AAMD Adaptive Behavior Scale– School Edition	PRO-ED
Adaptive Behavior Evaluation Scale	Hawthorne Educational Services
Independent Living Behavior Checklist	West Virginia Research and Training Center
Normative Adaptive Behavior Checklist	The Psychological Corporation
Scales of Independent Behavior	Bruininks, Woodcock, Weatherman, and Hill (1984)
Vineland Adaptive Behavior Scales	Sparrow et al. (1984)

indicate some limitations with the measures and emphasize that they should only be administered and interpreted by trained and experienced individuals.

3. □ Interview Schedules

Interviews traditionally constitute part of the assessment process within forensic assessments and have always been important means of collecting information about the personality, attitudes, and circumstances of the youth. However, in most cases interviews are conducted in informal and unsystematic ways. This is particularly interesting in light of the frequent finding that unstructured interviews constitute one of the poorest and most invalid means for collecting information in clinical, research, or institutional settings (Garb, 1989; Murphy & Davidshofer, 1988; Siassi, 1984).

There are, on the other hand, a number of more standardized interview schedules available, and there appear to be increasing efforts to evaluate and refine these through traditional psychometric procedures (Gutterman, O'Brien, & Young, 1987; Hodges, 1993). Table 5.7 identifies eight interview schedules designed for the collection of information from the youth or his or her parent. The format of these varies from highly structured to semistructured, with the latter allowing somewhat more latitude for the operation of clinical judgment.

Several of the instruments identified in the table are primarily designed as clinical instruments and are scored in terms of DSM-III-R or DSM-IV criteria. This includes the Child Assessment Schedule (CAS) (Hodges, 1985), the Diagnostic Interview for Children and Adolescents (Herjanic, Herjanic, Brown, & Wheatt, 1975), the Diagnostic Interview Schedule for Children (Costello, Edelbrock, Dulcan, Kalas, & Klaric, 1984), and the Revised Diagnostic Interview Schedule for Children (Shaffer, Schwab-Stone, Fisher, Cohen, Piacentini, Davies, et al., 1993). We will discuss the DSM-IV diagnostic system in a later chapter but will make some comments at this point on this type of measure.

Table 5.7. □ Standardized Interview Schedules

Measure	Source/reference
Adolescent Drug Abuse Diagnosis Instrument	Friedman and Utada (1989)
Adolescent Problem Inventory	Freedman et al. (1978)
Child Assessment Schedule	Hodges (1985)
Diagnostic Interview for Children	Costello et al. (1984)
Diagnostic Interview Schedule for Children and Adolescents	Herjanic et al. (1975)
Interview for Antisocial Behavior	Kazdin and Esveldt-Dawson (1986)
Psychopathy Checklist	Hare (1991)
Revised Diagnostic Interview Schedule for Children and Adolescents	Shaffer et al. (1993)
Semistructured Clinical Interview for Children	McConaughy and Achenbach (1990)

The CAS (Hodges, 1985; Hodges, Cools, & McKnew, 1989) is representative of these clinical instruments. This interview schedule provides for a systematic and comprehensive assessment of the youth's psychological functioning. The first part of the instrument consists of a set of structured questions directed to the youth and dealing with a wide variety of issues relating to behavior and functioning within the home, school, and community environments. Detailed guidance is given regarding the conduct of the interview and the scoring of responses. The second part of the interview requires the examiner to summarize his or her clinical observations from the interview.

The CAS is scored in terms of a set of Symptom Complex Scales that correspond to the diagnostic categories represented in DSM-III-R (e.g., "attention deficit with hyperactivity"; "overanxious disorder"; "oppositional defiant disorder"). It also yields scores reflecting the youth's level of adaptation within various areas. The interview schedule was designed for use by clinicians, but it may also be used by nonclinicians with some training in administration of the instrument.

As we indicated, there is now considerable research activity being conducted in connection with these structured clinical interviews (Gutterman et al., 1987; Hodges, 1993). There remains, however, some controversy over their psychometric properties. In particular, questions have been raised about the reliability of diagnoses yielded by the instruments and about the construct validity of the psychiatric categories represented in the instruments (see, e.g., Last, 1987; Werry, 1992). We will return to these issues later in the book.

The Semistructured Clinical Interview for Children (McConaughy & Achenbach, 1990) forms, as we have seen, part of the Child Behavior Checklist family of instruments. Other interview schedules identified in Table 5.7 are designed for assessing a variety of antisocial attitudes and behaviors. They include the Adolescent Drug Abuse Diagnosis Interview (Friedman & Utada, 1989), the Adolescent

Problem Inventory (Freedman, Rosenthal, Donahoe, Schlundt, & McFall, 1978), the Interview for Antisocial Behavior (Kazdin & Esveldt-Dawson, 1986), and the Psychopathy Checklist (Hare, 1991). The latter instrument is discussed further in Chapter 7.

4. □ Other Types of Personality and Behavioral Measures

There are two other types of personality and behavioral assessment measures that may sometimes have utility within juvenile justice settings. One category includes projective instruments such as the Children's Apperception Test and the Rorschach. These must be used by a trained clinician with special training in administration and scoring of the instruments.

Another group of instruments include structured observation schedules. Examples of these include the Direct Observation Form (Achenbach, 1991b) and the Classroom Observation Code (Abikoff & Gittelman, 1985). These often represent valid means of collecting information about behavioral adjustment. The drawback, of course, is that they are relatively time-consuming means for collecting behavioral information. Mash and Terdal (1988) and Sattler (1992) provide further discussions of these two categories of instruments.

5. □ Measures of Attitudes, Values, and Beliefs

We had earlier indicated considerable theoretical and empirical support for the hypothesis that attitudes, values, and beliefs are intimately involved in criminal activity. As such, they constitute important considerations in a wide range of judicial assessments, including risk and need levels. Table 5.8 identifies a number

Table 5.8. □ Measures of Attitudes, Values, and Beliefs

Measure	Source/reference
Attitudes Toward Institutional Authority	Rigby (1982)
Attitude Toward Legal Agencies	Shaw and Wright (1967)
Attitude Toward Probation Officers	Shaw and Wright (1967)
Criminal Sentiments Scale	Gendreau et al. (1979)
Neutralization Scale	Shields and Whitehall (1994)
Pride in Delinquency Scale	Shields and Whitehall (1991)
Revised Legal Attitudes Questionnaire	Kravitz, Cutler, and Brock (1993)

of attitudinal instruments that are the subject of current research and clinical attention.

The Criminal Sentiments Scale (Gendreau, Grant, Leipciger, & Collins, 1979) is an example of this type of instrument. This self-report measure contains 41 items and yields three subscores relating to different aspects of criminal behavior:

1. Attitudes toward laws, courts, and police
2. Tolerance for law violations
3. Identification with criminal others

The scale requires at least a grade 6 reading ability, but it may also be presented in an interview format. Information on the psychometric properties of the scale have been presented by Shields and Simourd (1991) and Simourd (in press). A related instrument is the Pride in Delinquency Scale (Shields & Whitehall, 1991), which is designed to assess the youth's attitudes toward engagement in various criminal activities. The scale asks the respondent to indicate the degree to which he or she would experience pride or shame in committing specific criminal acts (e.g., "beating up a child molester," "selling cocaine," "seeing a store being robbed and not calling the police"). Shields and Simourd (1991) and Simourd (in press) have presented some preliminary psychometric data for this instrument.

Brodsky and Smitherman's (1983) earlier review of forensically relevant instruments includes a number of other attitudinal measures appropriate for use with young offenders. One limitation to be noted in connection with these measures is that, in general, less psychometric data are available for them than for the established standardized personality and behavioral measures. However, there are increased calls for attention to these attitudinal and cognitive variables (e.g., Andrews & Bonta, 1994; Guerra, Huesmann, & Hanish, 1994; Hawkins et al., 1992; Hoge, et al., 1994), and more research may be expected in the future.

6. □ The Role of Personality, Behavioral, and Attitudinal Measures in Juvenile Justice Systems

There are a number of areas of forensic decision making in which information about personality, behavioral, or attitudinal characteristics of the youth is relevant, and, in fact, inferences about these characteristics are commonly observed in the processing of offenders. On the other hand, and as we have seen, the inferences and judgments about the youth's personality, behavior, or attitudes are generally based on informal interviews and observations, and their reliability and validity is often questionable. Use of the standardized instruments described in this chapter will, we feel, enhance the quality of these inferences and the decisions based on them.

Scores from these measures are, for example, relevant to judgments about aggravating and mitigating conditions: Severe emotional or behavioral disorder is often considered a mitigating factor in assessing the seriousness of a criminal act and in making both preadjudicatory and postadjudicatory decisions. Instruments such as the MMPI-A, the Revised Behavior Problem Checklist, and the Basic Personality Inventory yield objective information about these dimensions. On the other hand, crimes committed in association with antisocial and procriminal attitudes are often considered more serious than those committed in the absence of such attitudes. The attitudinal measures described here may, therefore, be useful in forming judgments about aggravating conditions.

These instruments also have role to play in judgments about mental maturity or competency, which are, in turn, related to decisions about competency to stand trial, ability to consent to treatment, waivers, and other issues. As we have seen, several of the personality tests and interview schedules identified in this chapter are specifically designed to yield scores corresponding to psychiatric categories relevant to those judgments. Included are the MMPI-A, the Psychopathy Checklist, and the interview schedules yielding DSM-IV diagnoses. We will discuss these further in Chapter 7. In addition, the standardized measures of adaptive functioning yield scores reflective of mental maturity or competency.

Risk assessment constitutes another area in which scores from these personality, behavioral, and attitudinal instruments have a contribution to make. As we showed earlier, there is ample support for the position that certain personality, behavioral, and attitudinal characteristics are associated with increased risk for criminal activity. In fact, several of the instruments reviewed this chapter have been specifically related to indices of criminal activity. Examples include the Revised Behavior Problem Checklist, the Basic Personality Inventory, and the MMPI-A.

These standardized instruments also have an important role to play in judgments of criminogenic needs and responsivity, which, in turn, may impact on a variety of preadjudicatory and postadjudicatory decisions. We had earlier argued that the assessment of criminogenic need factors should form an important element within the juvenile justice system. This conclusion is explicit within the General Personality and Social Psychological Model of Criminal Conduct (Andrews & Bonta, 1994; Andrews et al., 1990), which stresses the necessity for carefully identifying and targeting factors that are associated with criminal activity and are amenable to change. The behavioral and attitudinal measures are particularly important in this respect. The identification of specific dysfunctional behaviors and attitudes enables one to focus on meaningful targets for intervention.

The model also stresses the importance of assessing responsivity factors within the youth. We know that youths react differently to different treatments, whether periods of incarceration, a form of counseling, or whatever. Some of the personality, behavioral, and attitudinal scales can be useful in guiding those decisions. For example, the knowledge that a youth holds essentially prosocial rather than antisocial attitudes can be an important consideration in deciding the type of counseling to offer. Similarly, information from a behavioral measure that the youth has a propensity for violent and sadistic acts might affect the nature of the imposed custody. The instruments have a similar role to play in judgments about amenability to treatment.

Although we feel that these instruments have important uses in the assessment of young offenders, there are two cautions noted in our discussion that we wish to stress. First, some of these instruments, particularly the personality tests, involve rather complex scoring and interpretation procedures. A high level of expertise is often required for their use. Their application is somewhat facilitated by the increasing availability of computerized scoring and interpretation protocols, but even here knowledge about personality assessment is important.

The second caution relates to the limitations we have noted in connection with the psychometric properties of the instruments. We have indicated that most of the instruments identified in this chapter demonstrate adequate levels of reliability and validity. Still, there are limits in this respect, and it is important for practitioners to familiarize themselves with whatever limits exist for the specific instruments they intend to employ. We will discuss these issues further in Chapter 8.

Chapter 6

□

Assessing Environmental Factors

Mental health professionals have traditionally focused on personality and behavioral characteristics in their assessments of young offenders. For various reasons, the environment in which the youth is functioning has been relatively ignored. We now know that this is an error. Psychological research and theory have demonstrated conclusively that a full understanding of child development and behavior can only be achieved when consideration is given to the total environment in which the child is functioning (Bronfenbrenner, 1979, 1986). This total environment includes the child's relations with parents, dynamics of the larger family environment, the peer group, the school, and the community in which the child is living.

We have also seen that the most recent theory and research on the causes of youthful offending has stressed the importance of family, peer, and community factors (see, e.g., Andrews et al., 1992; Elliott et al., 1985; Henggeler, 1991; Loeber & Stouthamer-Loeber, 1986; Yoshikawa, 1994). We do not always have a full understanding of the processes whereby these factors influence deviant behavior, but it is clear, for example, that assessments of risk for criminal activity are enhanced when aspects of family functioning are taken into consideration (e.g., Blaske, Borduin, Henggeler, & Mann, 1989; Hoge et al., 1994).

The importance of environmental factors receives explicit recognition in Child Welfare types of judicial models, particularly those guided by integrated theories such as the General Personality and Social Psychological Model of Criminal Conduct (Andrews & Bonta, 1994; Andrews et al., 1990). Thus, in many systems there is an explicit acknowledgment that interventions in the family, peer, and community environment are essential for truly effective juvenile justice interventions. It is more often the case, however, that these factors receive informal consideration in the processing of youthful offenders and, in many cases, are taken into account even where official policy presumably excludes their consideration. An example is Hoge, Andrews, and Leschied's (1995) demonstration that factors relating to the home environment affected decisions about referrals to custody in a system in which policy dictated that these referrals be based solely on factors related to the nature of criminal activity. This problem arises particularly in situations when there is some ambiguity about the social welfare role of the juvenile justice system (Markwart, 1992).

Whether implicit or explicit, there are many cases in which inferences about the youth's home and community situation are involved in judicial decisions. As is usually the case, however, these inferences are generally based on informal and unsystematic assessment procedures. There are, on the other hand, standardized instruments available for collecting this information. We will consider in this chapter measures of family and parental functioning, school performance, and peer group associations.

There is another type of environmental measure that we will also consider later in the chapter. This focuses on the correctional or treatment environment provided for the youth. The need for standardized tools for assessing the treatment environment has long been recognized in research and evaluation contexts: Our ability to evaluate the effectiveness of our interventions depends very heavily on our ability to objectively describe the interventions. We also believe that systematic descriptions of program options have a role to play in decisions about individual offenders. If we are truly interested in achieving an optimal match between the needs and responsivity characteristics of offenders and the sanction or treatment provided them, then it is important to have some means for describing the sanctions and treatments. We will consider some representative measures later in the chapter and also explore more fully the role of these measures in judicial processing.

1. □ Measures of Family Functioning and Parenting

Our focus in this section is on standardized measures designed for assessing aspects of the family environment. The first group of instruments focus on the total family environment, while the second provides for a more specific focus on parental practices and parent–child relations. We will consider only self-report and interview instruments. Other types of measures, including observation schedules and projective techniques, are described by Jacob and Tennenbaum (1988), L'Abate and Bagarozzi (1993), and Touliatos, Perlmutter, and Straus (1990).

Table 6.1 identifies six standardized measures of family functioning. All are self-report measures designed for completion by parents and, in some cases, the youth. While the nature of the constructs vary across the instruments, all are capable of providing useful information about family functioning.

The Family Environment Scale (Moos & Moos, 1986) serves as an example of this type of instrument. This 90-item self-report measure is designed to provide a broad assessment of family functioning in a variety of family types, including single-parent families, step-families, and foster families. The instrument is scored in terms of 10 subscales, listed in Table 6.2. Each describes a different aspect of

Table 6.1. □ Measures of Family Functioning

Measure	Source/reference
Family Adaptability and Cohesion Evaluation	Olson, Partner, and Lavoie (1985)
Family Assessment Device	Epstein, Baldwin, and Bishop (1983)
Family Assessment Measure III	Multihealth Systems
Family Beliefs Inventory	Roehling and Robin (1986)
Family Environment Scale	Moos and Moos (1986)
Family Events Checklist	Patterson, Reid and Dishion (1992)

family functioning. For example, the cohesion subscale represents the degree of support that family members provide for one another, while the control subscale describes the degree to which rules and procedures are followed within the family. Billings and Moos (1982) have also developed a typology of family types from the measure. This typology characterizes the family in terms of its overall orientation. Two of the family types, conflict-oriented and disorganized, are often encountered in juvenile justice contexts.

A valuable feature of the Family Environment Scale relates to the availability of normative data for both normal and dysfunctional families. These data are particularly important when dealing with the type of problem family from which many delinquents come. Moos and Moos (1986) also report a number of analyses supportive of the reliability and validity of the Family Environment Scale. It must be kept in mind, though, that scores from the instrument represent family member's *perceptions* of family functioning rather than direct information about functioning. On the other hand, these perceptions are often the most important considerations in placement and treatment decisions.

Table 6.3 presents examples of another type of instrument, which provides a specific focus on parenting practices and parent–child relations. One of these instruments, the Parenting Risk Scale, involves a structured interview format, while the others entail rating, checklist, or questionnaire formats.

Table 6.2. □ Subscales for the Family Environment Scale

Cohesion	Intellectual-cultural orientation
Expressiveness	Active-recreational orientation
Conflict	Moral-religious emphasis
Independence	Organization
Achievement orientation	Control

Source: Moos and Moos (1986).

Table 6.3. □ Measures of Parenting

Measure	Source/reference
Children's Report of Parental Behavior Inventory	Schluderman and Schluderman (1970)
Parent–Adolescent Relationship Questionnaire	Robin, Koepke, and Moye (1990)
Parent Practices Scale	Strayhorn and Weidman (1988)
Parenting Risk scale	Mrazek, Mrazek, and Klinnert (1995)
Weinberger Parenting Inventory	Feldman and Weinberger (1994)

The Children's Report of Parental Behavior Inventory is representative of this type of measure. The instrument was developed by Schluderman and Schluderman (1970, 1983) from Schaefer's (1965) earlier analyses of parental behavior. The self-report measure was originally designed for completion by the youth, but it may also be completed by parents. The measure is scored in terms of three factor scores representing different dimensions of parenting: acceptance/rejection, psychological control/psychological autonomy, and firm control/lax control. These are, in fact, dimensions of parenting that have been implicated in criminal activity in young people. Some reliability and validity data are available for the measure (Schluderman & Schluderman, 1970, 1983).

2. □ Measures of School Performance and Adjustment

The achievement tests discussed in Chapter 4 provide important means for objectively assessing the youth's academic performance relative to his or her developmental level. In addition, teachers constitute an important source of information about the performance and behavior of the youth in school. This is particularly true when they are provided with appropriate tools for expressing the assessments (Hoge, 1983; Hoge & Coladarci, 1989). Relevant to this are some of the teacher-completed behavioral checklists and rating scales identified in Chapter 5 that provide scores reflecting classroom adjustment. For example, the Revised Behavior Problem Checklist (Quay & Peterson, 1987) yields scores reflecting conduct-disordered behavior in the classroom setting. Similar scores are also available from the parent and teacher versions of Achenbach's (1991a, 1991b) Child Behavior Checklist. The teacher version of this instrument also provides for the collection of information on academically relevant motivation, attitudes, and performance levels. The self-concept measures reviewed Chapter 5 may also contribute useful information regarding the youth's attitudes and values regarding educational issues. We will also see in Chapter 7 some of the broad-based risk assessment instruments that permit the collection of information regarding academic performance and school adjustment.

There are also measures designed specifically for assessing the youth's attitudes and values regarding schooling issues. Table 6.4 identifies a sampling of these instruments. The Student Attitude Measure (Butler, Novy, Kagan, & Gates, 1994) is representative of this type of measure. This self-report measure yields information about the youth's perceptions of his or her educational experience in a number of dimensions, including motivation for academic achievement, confidence in abilities, feelings of mastery over the school environment, and ability to evaluate one's own work. Most of these instruments have been developed for research purposes, but when used with some caution they are capable of providing useful information in clinical settings.

3. □ Measures of Peer Group Associations

As we have seen, the nature of the youth's peer friendships and associations constitutes an important consideration in assessing the situation of the youth. Information about these associations is usually collected through interviews with parents, teachers, or childcare workers or through informal observations of the youth in community settings.

On the other hand, standardized assessments also have a role to play in this respect. For example, some of the behavioral checklists and rating scales reviewed in Chapter 5 provide direct information about peer group experiences. Achenbach's (1991a) Child Behavior Checklist provides an illustration. The instrument contains a number of items reflecting peer group associations (e.g., "bad companions," "prefers young friends," "prefers older friends") as well as factor scores relevant to peer relations (e.g., withdrawn, social problems, aggressive behavior). In addition, certain of the self-concept measures described in Chapter 5 provide indices of the youth's perceptions of his or her peer group experiences. We will also

Table 6.4. □ Measures of Educational Attitudes

Measure	Source/reference
Comprehensive Assessment Program: School Attitude Measure (2nd ed.)	American Testronics
Minnesota School Attitude Survey	SRA
School Interest Inventory	Riverside Publishing
Student Attitude Measure	Butler et al. (1994)
Survey of School Attitudes	The Psychological Corporation

see in Chapter 7 how some of the broad-based risk assessment instruments attempt to take account of negative peer group associations.

4. □ Measures of Correctional and Therapeutic Environments

Table 6.5 lists four standardized measures suitable for assessing correctional and community treatment environments. These instruments have been used primarily as research and evaluation tools, but as we indicated, they may also be employed in assessment and in decisions relating to the youthful offender. We will discuss these uses later.

Two of those instruments are drawn from the set of Social Climate Scales developed by Moos: the Correctional Institutions Environment Scale (Moos, 1986a) and the Community-Oriented Programs Environment Scale (Moos, 1986b). These instruments contain 90–100 true–false items, and they are designed for completion by program staff, participants, or residents. Scores from the instruments provide information about a number of program dimensions, including structure, staff attitudes, staff–client relationships, and goal clarity. Considerable information about the reliability and validity of the instruments is presented in the manuals.

The Prison Environment Inventory (Wright, 1985) represents another measure of the climate of correctional institutions. This 48-item scale is scored in terms of seven factor scores: program structure, emotional feedback, social climate, staff support, activity planning, safety, and privacy. While these dimensions do have some face validity, it must be acknowledged that only limited support for the reliability and validity of the instrument are as yet available.

The fourth instrument listed in the table, the Correctional Program Assessment Inventory (Gendreau & Andrews, 1994), is a relatively new instrument, and, as yet, little research on its psychometric properties are available. The instrument is designed as an aid in describing and assessing correctional environments. The measure is completed on the basis of information about program characteristics

Table 6.5. □ Measures of Correctional and Therapeutic Environments

Measure	Source/reference
Community-Oriented Programs Environment Scale	Moos (1986b)
Correctional Institutions Environment Scale	Moos (1986a)
Correctional Program Assessment Inventory	Gendreau and Andrews (1994)
Prison Environment Inventory	Wright (1985)

collected through interviews, observations, or checklists. It yields scores in the following areas: program implementation, client preservice assessment, program characteristics, therapeutic integrity, relapse prevention, staff characteristics, and research and evaluation.

The Correctional Program Assessment Inventory provides a description of program characteristics in these areas, but it is also designed to indicate the quality or integrity of correctional programming. This assessment of quality is made in terms of the General Personality and Social Psychological Model of Criminal Conduct (Andrews & Bonta, 1994; Andrews et al., 1990) described earlier. While the instrument was originally developed for use in adult correctional settings, Hoge et al. (1995) have provided an example of its application to juvenile correctional settings.

5. □ The Role of Environmental Assessments in Juvenile Justice Systems

The standardized measures of family functioning and parenting have, we feel, an important role to play in assessing the youthful offender. As we saw earlier, family dynamics and parenting have been clearly implicated as causal factors in youthful offending. To this extent, measures focusing on specific aspects of family dysfunction, abuse, and parenting deficits are critical in the formation of risk, need, and responsivity judgments and, in turn, in decisions about placement and programming. This is particularly true, of course, in systems guided by a child welfare or rehabilitation model. There are also circumstances in which the family and parenting environment is relevant to the consideration of mitigating factors, and the measures would play a role here as well.

The importance of assessing family factors is reinforced by recent research demonstrating the effectiveness of interventions with high-risk youth that directly target aspects of family and parental functioning. Good illustrations of this work may be found in the research of Henggeler and his colleagues (Borduin, Mann, Cone, Henggeler, Fricci, Blaske, et al., 1995; Henggeler, Melton, & Smith, 1992; Henggeler, Melton, Smith, Schoenwald, & Hanley, 1993) demonstrating the effectiveness of such interventions with high-risk youths that directly target aspects of family and parental functioning. There is growing evidence that these interventions are superior to those that focus only on the youth.

There are, on the other hand, some particular cautions to be noted with these measures of family functioning and parenting. While the various instruments listed in Tables 6.1 and 6.3 are generally well established and more or less extensively researched, questions sometimes remain about their psychometric properties, particularly with reference to construct validity. Characterizing family dynamics and parenting practices is a very difficult matter, and the meaningfulness of the constructs yielded by the instruments is sometimes less than clear (Holden & Edwards, 1989; L'Abate & Bagarozzi, 1993). On the other hand, even given this caution, standardized instruments with explicit operational definitions remain preferable to the informal and unsystematic assessments of family and parenting characteristics generally observed in juvenile justice settings.

Similar points may be made with respect to the standardized measures yielding information about school adjustment and performance and peer group associations. These are critical variables in the assessment of young offenders, and the use of standardized instruments with known psychometric properties is preferable to the informal and unsystematic data collection procedures so often observed.

Measures of correctional and therapeutic environments was another type of instrument we considered in this chapter. These measures have been used primarily for research and evaluation purposes. However, we have argued that they also have a role to play in juvenile decision making, particularly in placement and intervention decisions.

We have seen that placement decisions are often directed by security considerations. These involve, then, judgments of the level of risk represented by the youth. On the other hand, the actual placement would reflect judgments about the level of security represented in the various placement options. Instruments such as the Correctional Institutions Environment Scale and the Prison Environment Inventory provide objective means for assessing security levels.

The instruments also have a role to play in treatment decisions. There is a very sound theoretical and empirical basis for the assumption that the effectiveness of therapeutic interventions is enhanced when the characteristics of the client are carefully matched with features of the services provided (Beutler & Clarkin, 1990; Hoge & Andrews, 1986; Snow, 1991). We have already talked about the necessity for careful assessments of client responsivity characteristics in therapeutic decisions. The other side of this equation involves identifying features of the environment relevant to these responsivity characteristics. If we identify a youth as having marginal reading abilities, a need for a highly structured environment, and a high need for emotional support, then it is important to be able to identify environments in which these conditions would be accommodated.

We feel that the correctional and therapeutic environment measures discussed in this chapter have a role to play in these decisions. For example, the two measures of social climate developed by Moos (1986a,b)—the Correctional Institutions Environment Scale and the Community-Oriented Programs Environment Scale— are explicitly designed to assist in achieving an optimal match between characteristics of the offender and features of the setting in which they are to be placed. We will see another example of an assessment system incorporating both responsivity and environmental measures when we discuss the Conceptual Level Matching Model in the next chapter.

While the logic of a careful matching of client characteristics with environmental features is clear, it must be admitted that we are still limited in our ability to assess these environmental characteristics. Considerable evidence in support of the reliability and validity of the Correctional Institutions Environment Scale and the Prison Environment Inventory have been presented (Moos, 1986a,b), but there is still limited information available about the utility of those instruments in actual decision situations. There is even less information about the other two instruments included in Table 6.5. They must continue to be regarded as experimental tools at the present time.

Chapter 7

□

Diagnostic and Classification Systems

The previous three chapters contained reviews of individual measuring instruments, all of which yield scores reflecting dimensions of aptitudes, personality, behavior, attitudes, or circumstances that are relevant in some way to juvenile justice decisions. The assessment tools and procedures considered in this chapter differ somewhat in that they provide information in the form of diagnostic scores directly relevant to forensic decisions. They are designed, in other words, to categorize the youth or to provide a diagnostic label that is directly linked to a judicial decision.

Reviews by Binder et al. (1988) and Quay (1987) reveal a long history of efforts to develop diagnostic and classification systems for adult and juvenile justice systems. However, these efforts have traditionally been viewed as relatively unsuccessful, with the systems yielding generally low levels of reliability and validity (Clemens, 1981; Megargee, 1977; Palmer, 1984). On the other hand, there has been considerable research activity in this area recently, and significant improvements in the quality of these efforts can be detected as demonstrated in reviews by Andrews and Bonta (1994), Champion (1994), Clements (1996), Van Voorhis (1994), and Wiebush, Baird, Krisberg, and Onek (1995). Much of this work focuses on the adult level, but there are, as we will see, developments relevant to the juvenile level as well.

Our discussion of these systems focuses on those that are the object of current research activity. We have divided them into categories reflecting the bases for the diagnoses or classifications:

- Personality-based diagnostic systems
- Behaviorally based diagnostic systems
- Offense-based risk systems
- Broad-based risk/need systems

1. □ Personality-Based Diagnostic Systems

Four systems are identified in Table 7.1 that have as their foundation personality traits or characteristics. All four of these have seen wide application in juvenile justice systems and all are the subject of current research activity.

Table 7.1. ☐ Personality-Based Diagnostic Systems

Measure	Reference/source
Conceptual Level Matching Model (CLMM)	Reitsma-Street and Leschied (1988)
Diagnostic and Statistical Manual of Mental Disorders, Fourth Edition (DSM-IV)	American Psychiatric Association (1994)
Interpersonal Maturity Level Classification System (I-Level)	Warren (1983)
Minnesota Multiphasic Personality Inventory (MMPI)	National Computer Systems

1.1. ☐ Diagnostic and Statistical Manual of Mental Disorders, Fourth Edition (DSM-IV)

DSM-IV is the official diagnostic system of the psychiatric profession (American Psychiatric Association, 1994). The manual presents definitions of various categories of mental disorder, with the categories defined in terms of specific diagnostic criteria. Information about the etiology, prevalence, and developmental progression of the disorders is also presented. The diagnostic categories within the system are frequently utilized by mental health professionals in assessments of young offenders and are sometimes used in official judicial processing activities. In fact, the diagnostic system is sometimes regarded as the unofficial mental health nomenclature system of the judicial system.

DSM-IV represents the latest version of the diagnostic system. It includes two sets of diagnostic categories, one applicable to children and adolescents and the other to adults. Age 18 is generally treated as the cut-off for adult diagnoses, and, hence, the categories from the child and adolescent section are most relevant to the youthful offender.

Table 7.2 identifies the diagnostic categories most relevant to the juvenile justice setting. The Conduct Disorder category includes in its diagnostic criteria criminal activities. However, other categories under the Attention Deficit and Disruptive Behavior Disorders are also frequently employed in assessing delinquents. DSM-IV also includes provision for diagnosing cognitive, perceptual, and academic deficits, and these are also sometimes relevant in juvenile justice decisions.

The actual assessment of the DSM-IV categories has traditionally depended on structured or unstructured clinical interviews conducted by a mental health professional. However, and as noted in Chapter 5, efforts are being made to develop more systematic assessment tools that will yield DSM-IV diagnoses. For example, certain personality tests, including MMPI-A and the Millon Adolescent Personality Inventory, yield scores corresponding to some of the diagnostic categories. Other efforts are being directed toward the development of standard-

Table 7.2. □ **Diagnostic Categories from DSM-IV Relevant to Young Offenders**

Attention-Deficit and Disruptive Behavior Disorders
  Attention-Deficit/Hyperactivity Disorder: Specific
  Attention-Deficit/Hyperactivity Disorder: Not Otherwise Specified
  Conduct Disorder
  Oppositional Defiant Disorder
  Disruptive Behavior Disorder

Source: American Psychiatric Association (1994).

ized inventory schedules designed to yield DSM-IV diagnoses. These were identified in Chapter 5, and we simply note here again that efforts to evaluate and refine these instruments are well underway (Gutterman et al., 1987; Hodges, 1993).

It should also be acknowledged that numerous criticisms have been advanced against the DSM-IV system, particularly as applied to children and adolescents (McReynolds, 1989; Quay, Routh, & Shapiro, 1987; Sattler, 1992). One criticism is that the system is based on rigid diagnostic categories rather than on personality or behavioral dimensions. Thus, either the child is diagnosed as conduct-disordered or as not conduct-disordered . A second criticism is that the diagnostic categories often do not reflect the latest research on these pathological conditions. Third, while explicit criteria are associated with the diagnostic categories, a high degree of clinical judgment is called for and levels of inter-rater agreement tend to be rather low. Finally, there is the criticism that the system is very reflective of a medical model and, hence, locates abnormal conditions within the individual placing little weight on environmental or social forces. It must be acknowledged that the latest version of the schedule, DSM-IV, includes efforts to address all of these criticisms, but problems still remain.

1.2. □ The Minnesota Multiphasic Personality Inventory (MMPI)

This is one of the most popular personality tests, and it, and its revised version, MMPI-2, continues to receive wide use in criminal justice settings. Most applications in these settings are based on a system for classifying offenders developed by Megargee (1984; Megargee & Bohn, 1979). This system is based on MMPI profiles, and it describes ten different offender types. The typology has been widely used as a basis for assessing risk levels and as a guide for treatment decisions. The classification system has been used and continues to be used with adolescents, although questions have been raised about its applicability at this level (see Vaneziano & Vaneziano, 1986; Zager, 1988).

Note should also be taken of MMPI-A, which represents a revision of the original MMPI, but with specific application to adolescents. It was developed in parallel with the recent creation of MMPI-2 and contains revised items, new standardization data, and new scoring procedures (Butcher, Williams, Graham, Archer, Tellegen, Ben-Porath, et al., 1992). A scoring format has also been proposed by Archer (1992), which yields considerable information about the personality and behavioral characteristics of the youth that might be useful in assessing risk, need, and responsivity levels. On the other hand, the new version has not been specifically applied to youthful offenders, and there is no evidence yet that the Megargee category system can be derived from the new version.

1.3. □ The Interpersonal Maturity Level Classification System (I-Level)

This system is based on a theory of personality that classifies individuals in terms of increasing levels of perceptual, cognitive, and interpersonal maturity. The system was adapted by Warren and her colleagues for the classification of adolescent delinquents (Warren, 1976), and the classification system has been widely used in juvenile justice systems as an aid in decision making, particularly with diversion and treatment decisions.

There are two levels of analysis represented in the I-Level system (Warren, 1976, 1983). The first entails describing the individual in terms of a continuum representing their social–perceptual frame of reference. The second stage entails a system for classifying the individual in terms of personality types derived from the above continuum. The nine empirically derived subtypes most relevant to the classification of young offenders are listed in Table 7.3.

Two methods for forming the classifications are available. The first involves an interview format, the CTPI-Level Interview (Warren, 1966), and the second is based on the Jesness Inventory (Jesness & Wedge, 1985), a self-report personality measure. The CTPI-I Level Interview is a 90-minute semistructured interview scored by means of a coding system. The major problem with the interview is that a detailed administration manual has not been published. Further, reliability and validity evaluations have generally yielded equivocal results (P. W. Harris, 1988).

The Jesness Inventory is a more highly developed measure as well as much more economical to administer. It is composed of 155 true–false items that can be understood with at least a grade 8 reading ability. Two sets of scores may be derived from the instrument. The first are based on a set of empirically derived personality scales, and the second is based on the nine personality types identified in Table 7.3.

Somewhat more evidence in support of the reliability and validity of the Jesness Inventory is available than for the interview instrument (P. W. Harris, 1988;

Table 7.3. □ **Categories from the I-Level System Relevant to Young Offenders**

I-Level	Category
I–2	Asocial passive
	Asocial aggressive
I 3	Immature conformist
	Cultural conformist
	Manipulator
I–4	Neurotic acting out
	Neurotic anxious
	Cultural identifier
	Situational-emotional reaction

Source: Warren (1976, 1983).

Jesness, 1988). Still, it must be acknowledged that only limited evidence exists regarding the predictive or dynamic validity of I-Level classification scores.

1.4. □ The Conceptual Level Matching Model (CLMM)

This is also a classification system designed as an aid in making placement and intervention decisions with young offenders. An additional feature of this model is that it attempts to characterize environments, and the ultimate goal is to achieve an optimal match between the characteristics of offender and environment. The current version of the model is based on Hunt's (1971) earlier research on conceptual level.

Individuals within this system are characterized in terms of their conceptual level. This refers very generally to the way in which they process information and approach tasks. Conceptual level and environmental type are each described in terms of four distinct categories. Optimal matches between conceptual level and environment are then identified. For example, the first conceptual level category describes an individual with a very concrete and egocentric orientation, and this is matched with a high-structure, high-support type of environment. A second category describes an independent, curious, cognitively complex individual; the ideal environment for this person would be one with low structure and cognitive challenges.

Assessing conceptual level and environmental structure is somewhat problematic. The former is typically assessed through the Paragraph Completion Method (Hunt, Butler, Noy, & Rosser, 1971), a semiprojective test that involves coding completed sentence stems. However, the manual for scoring the test is not widely available, and, further, there appears to be considerable controversy over the criteria to be employed in scoring (see Reitsma-Street & Leschied, 1988). It also appears that there is no standard basis for assessing environmental structure, although Moos' (1986a) Correctional Institutions Environment Scale and Wright's (1985) Prison Environment Inventory have been used under some circumstances.

The CLMM is a popular approach for many mental health professionals dealing with youthful offenders. Further, Reitsma-Street and Leschied's (1988) review revealed some support for the reliability and validity of applications of the model. On the other hand, evidence in support of the predictive validity of the instrument or its sensitivity to treatment effects (dynamic validity) is still somewhat limited.

2. □ Behaviorally Based Systems

These systems utilize patterns of observed behaviors as a basis for categorizing individuals. The most influential of these systems within juvenile justice settings has been the model developed by Quay (1964, 1966) out of earlier empirical research on pathological behaviors of children and adolescents. One version of this system is based on a fourfold classification system: inadequate–immature, unsocialized–subcultural, socialized–subcultural, and disturbed–neurotic. Each category describes a different type of delinquent, and the typology presumably has implications for placement and treatment decisions.

The assessment of these behavioral categories is generally based on one of two instruments, the Checklist for the Analysis of Life History Data or the Behavior Problem Checklist (Quay, 1964, 1966). The latter, as we saw earlier, is a behavioral checklist suitable for completion by parent, teacher, or clinician. Considerable research has been reported in connection with this classification system (Quay, 1987), and there is some support for reliability and validity. A delinquency typology has not yet been derived from the Revised Behavior Problem Checklist.

3. □ Offense-Based Risk Systems

Another group of instruments include those designed to provide estimates of the probability of future events. These are generally designed for predicting future criminal activity, violent criminal activity, or problems of institutional adjustment. They may also be employed in assessing the probability of general adjustment problems or of harm-to-self. This type of instrument is widely used in adult systems to aid in disposition and parole decisions, but it also may have utility in juvenile systems in which information about risk of continued offending is desired. As we saw in Chapter 2, risk assessments are often explicitly or implicitly involved in decisions about waivers or transfers, type of disposition, and the level of security to provide within custody settings.

Some risk instruments represent actuarial devices; that is, they were created through the empirical analysis of data-linking characteristics of offenders with incidences of criminal activity. These instruments generally provide a means for categorizing the individual (e.g., high, medium, low risk) or a statement of the probability that the individual will exhibit the predicted behavior (e.g., youths at this level have a 65% probability of reoffending within one year). Other instruments in this group are theoretically or clinically derived. However, these instruments generally do not meet the criteria for standardized psychological assessments.

Risk assessment measures may also be described in terms of the basis for the risk assessment. We will consider in this section those that are based primarily on offense-related factors. Another type of risk instrument is based on a broader range of predictor variables; we will consider this type in the next section.

Offense-based risk classification systems use information about the frequency and severity of prior and current offending as a basis for formulating predictions of future criminal activity. Other variables, such as age at first arrest, may also be included in the assessment. One example of such an instrument is the Salient Factor Score Index developed by the United States Parole Commission, which is widely utilized with adult offenders, although it could also be used with older juveniles. The six items in the scale reflect the offender's offense and incarceration history, age at current offense, and degree of drug dependence. Scores from the scale are expressed in terms of parole prognosis: poor, fair, good, very good.

A similar instrument developed specifically for juveniles is the North Dakota Risk Assessment Instrument. This is based on five factors: severity of the current offense, severity of prior adjudications, number of prior adjudications, age at first adjudication, and prior runaway behavior. The Colorado Security Placement Instrument shown in Figure 7.1 is an example of a risk instrument specifically developed to assess risk to self or others within the institutional setting. Other offense-based risk instruments are described by Champion (1994) and Wiebush et al. (1995).

These offense-based instruments do provide a systematic means for collecting information about the seriousness of prior and current criminal activity. Furthermore, there is evidence to indicate that these offense-based risk assessments have utility in the prediction of future behavior (Floud & Young, 1981; Champion, 1994). There are, however, three reservations to be stated in connection with these measures. First, while they do yield valid predictions of future behavior, levels of prediction are moderate and, hence, include significant numbers of false positive and negative predictions. Second, the range of predictive variables included in the instruments is quite narrow, limited as they are to factors relating to

Risk item		Score
1. Severity of Current Offense		___
Murder, rape, kidnap, escape	10	
Other violent	5	
All other	0	
2. Severity of Prior Adjudications		___
Violent offense	5	
Property offense	3	
Other/none	0	
3. Number of Prior Adjudications		___
Two or more	5	
Less than 2	0	
	Total Items 1–3	___

Total items 1–3. If score is 10 or higher, score as *secure placement*. If less than 10, score remaining stability items.

4. Age at First Referral		___
12–13	2	
14+	0	
5. History of Mental Health Outpatient Care		___
Yes	1	
No	0	
6. Youth Lived Alone or with Friends at Time of Current Adjudication		___
Yes	1	
No	0	
7. Prior Out-of-Home Placements		___
Yes	1	
No	0	
	Total items 1–7	___

Apply score to the following placement scale:
- 10+ Consider for secure
- 5–9 Short-Term Placement
- 0–4 Immediate Community Placement

Figure 7.1. □ The Colorado Security Placement Instrument

offense characteristics. As we saw in Chapter 1, the causes of criminal activity are complex and are probably poorly represented in this type of variable. This undoubtedly contributes to the relatively low level of prediction of these instruments. Third, to the extent that these offense-based instruments rely heavily on prior circumstances (e.g., number of prior convictions, severity of prior offending), they represent static variables and hence provide little guidance for intervention efforts.

4. □ Broad-Based Risk and Risk/Need Instruments

Another category of instruments includes those based on a broader range of variables. Some of these are designed to provide estimates of risk levels, and some are also designed to provide information about criminogenic needs. We had defined the latter as dynamic risk factors, that is, factors directly associated with criminal activity that are amenable to change and, if changed, reduce the chances of future criminal activity (Andrews & Bonta, 1994; Andrews et al., 1990). We will consider in this section several broad-based instruments that are the object of current research (see Table 7.4).

4.1. □ The Wisconsin Juvenile Probation and Aftercare Assessment Form

This instrument is representative of a number of risk and risk/need assessment instruments developed by state juvenile justice systems (see Champion, 1994; and Wiebush et al., 1995, for other examples). The instrument was developed by Baird (1981, 1985) from existing risk assessment instruments. The instrument is shown in Figure 7.2. The eight variables included in the scale reflect a range of both static (e.g., prior behavior) and dynamic (e.g., peer relationships) variables.

This measure has been widely adopted in juvenile justice systems and is being

Table 7.4. □ Broad-Based Risk/Need Assessment Instruments

Measure	Reference/source
Arizona Juvenile Risk Assessment Form	Ashford et al. (1986)
Firesetting Risk Interview	Kolko and Kazdin (1989)
Psychopathy Checklist–Revised	Multihealth Systems
Wisconsin Juvenile Probation and Aftercare Assessment Form	Baird (1981, 1985)
Youth Level of Service/Case Management Inventory	Hoge and Andrews (1994)

used as an aid in placement, classification, and other types of decisions. Unfortunately, there appear to be few assessments of the reliability or validity of the instrument. One exception is a study by Ashford and LeCroy (1988) that assessed the ability of the instrument to predict recidivism. The total score from the measure failed to significantly predict recidivism, and only one of the individual scores, age at first adjudication, showed a significant relation with the outcome variable.

4.2. ☐ The Arizona Juvenile Risk Assessment Form

Ashford, LeCroy, and Bond-Maupin (1986) developed this instrument to assist in aftercare decisions. The measure is similar to the Wisconsin measure, but it does contain a somewhat expanded range of risk variables, which include age, prior referrals, prior parole violations, runaway behavior, offense type, school, peer associations, alcohol/drug abuse, and family dynamics. Ashford and LeCroy (1990) assessed the predictive validity of this instrument. Both the total score and individual scores from the measure yielded predictions of recidivism significantly beyond chance levels. The most heavily weighted of the individual predictors were parole violations, arrest type, and family dynamics.

4.3. ☐ The Firesetting Risk Interview

This is a risk instrument with a very specific focus, assessing as it does the likelihood of firesetting activities. This parental interview schedule was developed by Kolko and Kazdin (1989) from a conceptual model of firesetting behavior. The model identifies 15 dimensions associated with this type of behavior; examples include curiosity about fire, early experience with fire, and level of parental supervision and control. Some data in support of the reliability and validity of the scale have been reported by Kolko and Kazdin (1989), but additional assessments of its psychometric properties are warranted.

4.4. ☐ The Psychopathy Checklist–Revised (PCL-R)

The PCL-R utilizes interview and file information to assess a range of traits and behaviors reflective of a psychopathic personality (Hare, 1991). The instrument was originally developed for use with adults, but it has been used successfully with young offenders (e.g., Forth, Hart, & Hare, 1990; Stanford, Ebner, Patton, & Williams, 1994). In addition, a version of the instrument specifically adapted for children and adolescents has been announced (Frick, O'Brien, Wooton, & McBurnett, 1994), although currently only limited information is available about the measure.

The PCL-R involves a semistructured interview format, with items within the format surveying a broad range of personality and behavioral dimensions, including lack of remorse or guilt, parasitic lifestyle, lack of realistic goals, and many short-term relationships. Certain items are modified when the scale is used with

Risk factor		Score
1. Age at First Adjudication		____
16 or older	0	
14 or 15	3	
13 or younger	5	
2. Prior Criminal Behavior		____
No prior arrests	0	
Prior arrest record; no formal sanctions	2	
Prior delinquency petitions sustained; no offenses classified as assaultive	3	
Prior delinquency petitions sustained; at least one assaultive offense recorded	5	
3. Institutional Commitments or Placements of 30 Days or More		____
None	0	
One	2	
Two or more	4	
4. Drug/Chemical Abuse		____
No known use or no interference with functioning	0	
Some disruption of functioning	2	
Chronic abuse or dependency	5	
5. Alcohol Abuse		____
No known use or no interference with functioning	0	
Occasional abuse, some disruption of functioning	1	
Chronic abuse, serious disruption of functioning	3	
6. Parental Control		____
Generally effective	0	
Inconsistent and/or ineffective	2	
Little or none	4	
7. School Displinary Problems		____
Attending, graduated, GED equivalence	0	
Problems handled at school level	1	
Severe truancy or behavioral problems	3	
Not attending/expelled	5	
8. Peer Relationships		____
Good support and influence	0	
Negative influence, companions involved in delinquent behavior	2	
Gang member	4	
TOTAL RISK SCORE		____

Source: Baird (1981, 1985).

Figure 7.2. □ Wisconsin Juvenile Probation and Aftercare Assessment of Risk Scale

adolescents (Forth et al., 1990). The scale yields a total score as well as two factor scores, one of which reflects psychopathic personality traits and the other a deviant, unstable lifestyle.

Considerable evidence in support of the reliability and validity of the instrument has been presented when used with adults (Hare, 1991). To the extent that scores from the instrument are predictive of recidivism, particularly violent recidivism, the instrument has an important role to play in risk and need assessments. While there is less information regarding the use of the measure with adolescents, the research reported by Forth et al. (1990), Frick et al. (1994), and Trevethan and Walker (1989) is promising.

4.5. □ The Youth Level of Service/Case Management Inventory (YLS/CMI)

This represents an adaptation of the Level of Service Inventory (LSI; Andrews & Bonta, 1994) for children and adolescents. The LSI is an instrument designed for assessing risk and need levels in adult offenders. It is normally completed on the basis of interviews with the client, reviews of file data and test scores, and any other information about the client. It is designed to be completed by mental health professionals and by frontline workers with training in the use of the instrument. The inventory has been widely adapted within justice and correctional systems as an aid in decision making, particularly probation and parole decisions. This was followed by the development of a youth version of the checklist, the Youth Level of Service Inventory, and, more recently, a version incorporating case management components, the YLS/CMI (Hoge & Andrews, 1994).

Table 7.5 outlines the six major components of the YLS/CMI. The first part of the measure consists of a set of 42 risk/need items identified in the research literature as related to juvenile criminal activity. These are divided into eight subscales: (1) prior and current offenses/dispositions (e.g., "prior custody"); (2) family circumstances/parenting (e.g., "inconsistent parenting"); (3) education/employment

Table 7.5. □ Components of the Youth Level of Service/Case Management Inventory

Part I	Assessment of risk/need factors
Part II	Summary of total and subscale risk/need scores
Part III	Other needs/special considerations
Part IV	Case manager's assessment of risk/need level
Part V	Placement recommendations
Part VI	Goals/case plan

Source: Hoge and Andrews (1994)

(e.g., "truancy"); (4) peer relations (e.g., "some delinquent friends"); (5) substance abuse (e.g., "chronic alcohol use"); (6) leisure/recreation (e.g., "no personal interests"); (7) personality/behavior (e.g., "short attention span"); and (8) attitudes/orientation (e.g., "callous, little concern for others"). The professional completing the form indicates whether or not the characteristic applies to the child. There is also an opportunity in this section to indicate areas of strength.

Part II of the instrument provides for the calculation of a total risk score as well as a graphic summary of scores across the eight risk/need areas. Figure 7.3 presents an example of a risk/need profile plotted against percentile scores based on a normative sample of adjudicated young male offenders (12–16 years old). This represents a hypothetical case of a high-risk youth.

Part III of the instrument allows for the assessment of a variety of other factors relevant to the youth. The latter includes characteristics of the youth or his or her circumstances that, while not directly linked to criminal activity, should be taken into account in case planning. Part IV permits the mental health provider to record his or her own estimate of risk and needs in the youth. Part V provides for an indication of the contact level recommended for the youth, and Part VI allows the professional to indicate a case management plan. This requires stating specific goals and means of achieving those goals.

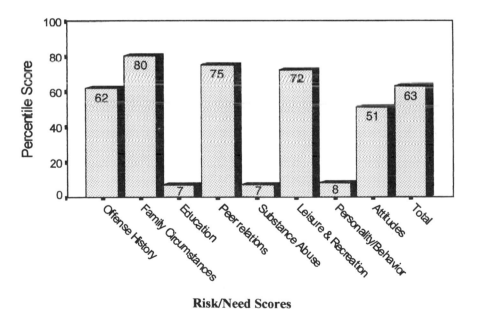

Risk/Need Scores

Figure 3. □ Example of a risk/need profile from Part II of the YLS/CMI.

There are several potential strengths associated with the YLS/CMI. First, it provides for a very broad assessment of factors known to be associated with youth crime. The selection of items in Part I was based on a review of the most current theoretical and empirical literature on the causes of youthful criminal activity. Second, the inventory provides direct information about need areas in the client, that is, areas in which interventions would be appropriate. Third, the instrument provides a systematic basis for collecting information relevant to aggravating and mitigating circumstances. Fourth, the instrument is designed for completion by probation officers and other frontline workers with some training. Finally, the detailed information about clients and their circumstances is of value from a management information point of view.

The YLS/CMI is a relatively new instrument for which only preliminary psychometric data are available (Hoge & Andrews, 1994, 1996). However, considerable psychometric support is available for the two instruments on which the inventory is based, the LSI (Andrews & Bonta, 1995) and the Youth Level of Service Inventory (Andrews, Robinson, & Hoge, 1984; Simourd, Hoge, Andrews, & Leschied, 1994).

5. ☐ Other Diagnostic Instruments

There are a number of other forensically relevant diagnostic assessment instruments that bear mention, although in most cases their relevance to the juvenile justice setting has not yet been established.

One of these instruments is the Sentencing Factors Inventory (Andrews, Robblee, Saunders, Huartson, Robinson, Kiessling, et al., 1987), which is designed to provide a standardized assessment of high-consensus aggravating and mitigating circumstances. Included in the inventory are items assessing the nature of the crime, the circumstances surrounding its occurrence, impact on the victim, and the offender's conduct following the offense. The authors have presented some preliminary psychometric data in support of the instrument when used with adult offenders, and it could be easily adapted to the juvenile justice setting.

Another group of standardized forensic instruments focus specifically on assessments of competency to stand trial. These include the Competency to Stand Trial Assessment Instrument (Weisstub, 1984) and the Fitness Interview Test (Roesch, Webster, & Eaves, 1984). Grisso's (1986) review reveals, however, numerous limitations of these efforts. Furthermore, as yet none of these instruments has been adapted for the juvenile level. Note might, however, be made of the Competence Assessment for Standing Trial for Defendants with Mental Retardation (Everington & Dunn, 1995). This instrument may have some utility with developmentally delayed adolescents.

6. ☐ The Role of Diagnostic and Classification Systems in Juvenile Justice Systems

The systems reviewed in this section have relevance for the entire range of decision categories represented in juvenile justice systems. Their application is somewhat different than that of the individual instruments reviewed earlier in that these systems have been designed specifically for application to forensic decision making. We will consider the issue of relevance first in connection with the personality and behavior based diagnostic systems.

6.1. ☐ Personality- and Behaviorally Based Systems

The assessment systems discussed under this heading are all designed to yield scores reflecting diagnostic categories such as socialized aggressive, conduct disordered, or passive conformist. These instruments have been widely used in juvenile justice settings. For example, they are often employed as aids in judgments about aggravating and mitigating factors and of mental status and mental maturity. They are utilized in this case to provide information about levels of cognitive and emotional maturity. The *DSM-IV* system is particularly relevant in this connection since it provides specific guidelines for assessing levels of maturity in these areas.

These personality and behaviorally based systems are also capable of providing valuable information about criminogenic needs, responsivity levels, and amenability to treatment. In fact, all of the systems provide for systematic links between diagnostic categories and treatments. For example, the CLMM provides relatively precise guidelines for matching delinquents with varying cognitive styles with therapeutic environments (Reitsma-Street & Leschied, 1988). Similarly, the MMPI-A has long been used as a basis for guiding intervention decisions with disturbed and antisocial adolescents (Archer, 1989).

The personality and behaviorally based systems also have a role to play in risk assessments, although, as we will see, other types of risk and risk/need assessment tools are probably more useful in this connection. In any case, general levels of risk for antisocial activity may be derived from all of the systems reviewed. For example, certain MMPI-A profiles have been associated with heightened risk for substance abuse (Archer, 1989), while the I-Level classification system has been shown to have utility in predicting criminal and other antisocial activity (Jesness & Wedge, 1984).

While these systems continue to be widely used in juvenile justice systems, there are some general reservations to be stated. First, reliability remains a concern with some of these systems, particularly *DSM-IV* and CLMM. Second, the construct validity of many of the diagnostic categories represented in these systems is problematic; examples of this point were noted in connection with the *DSM-IV* system. Third, there still remains limited information about the dynamic or treatment validity of these diagnostic systems; there are, in fact, relatively few systematic demonstrations that different types of treatment work differentially with different diagnostic categories. Finally, there is the issue we have raised before of the degree of correspondence between psychological and legal constructs. A designation of low cognitive and emotional maturity from the CLMM interview may not be consistent with a legal definition of diminished responsibility.

6.2. □ Offense-Based Risk Systems

Instruments of this type are designed to yield predictions about future antisocial or self-destructive behaviors. As such, they are widely used as an aid in forming risk judgments that are, in turn, employed in diversion, disposition, and placement decisions. The measures are particularly important in systems reflecting a crime-control type of model, where risk for future criminal activity is a primary concern. However, they have a role to play in other types of systems wherever there is a concern for the likelihood of future antisocial or self-destructive behavior.

Our earlier discussion of these instruments suggested that some caution be exercised in utilizing these measures for forensic decisions. First, there is relatively little information about the predictive validity of these instruments when used with juvenile offenders. Second, the validity information available for adult versions of these measures suggests that they have limited predictive value (Andrews & Bonta, 1994). Finally, and as we noted before, because these instruments are based largely on historical or static variables, they provide only limited information regarding criminogenic need or responsivity and, hence, can provide little guidance regarding intervention efforts.

6.3. □ Broad-Based Risk and Risk/Need Systems

This category includes measures that provide a broader assessment of risk and risk/need variables than any of the other types of instruments. The ability of these instruments to provide a broad picture of the youth's characteristics and circumstances means that they can be of great value in the formation of the entire range of judgments involved in forensic decisions.

While the information is limited at present, there is growing evidence that these broad-based instruments have value in assessing risk for future antisocial activities. This was demonstrated in the Ashford and LeCroy (1990) study in which the Arizona Juvenile Risk Assessment Form showed superior predictive validity compared with a risk instrument based solely on offense-based factors. We also note in this connection that considerable support for the predictive validity of adult versions of the YLS/CMI and PCL-R instruments has appeared (Hare, 1991; Andrews & Bonta, 1995). A major value of these latter instruments is the incorporation of items measuring the youth's attitudes, values, and beliefs regarding criminal activity. As we have seen, this type of variable is closely linked with youth crime, and its inclusion in these measures likely enhances their predictive power.

Instruments such as the Arizona Juvenile Risk Assessment Form (Ashford et al., 1986) and the YLS/CMI (Hoge & Andrews, 1994) provide very complete pictures of the personality, behavioral, attitudinal, and circumstantial characteristics of the young person, and thus, have great potential value in forming judgments about aggravating and mitigating factors, as well as about mental status. A similar argument may be made for the PCL-R (Hare, 1991).

We have also suggested that the broad-based risk/need instruments have a particularly important role to play in placement and treatment decisions. This is especially evident where a General Personality and Social Psychological Model of Criminal Conduct (Andrews & Bonta, 1994; Andrews et al., 1990) type of model is accepted. The assumption is that interventions with youthful offenders will be successful to the extent that they target actual criminogenic needs and take account of meaningful responsivity factors. The strength of these broad-based instruments is that they have the potential for providing this type of information.

There are some cautions to be stated regarding the broad-based instruments. First, it must be acknowledged that the reliability and validity of the procedures, when used with children and adolescents, have not been thoroughly investigated. Considerable support does exist for the predictive validity of adult versions of some of these instruments, but this should not be generalized to the adolescent level. Second, these broad-based measures depend upon information about the client collected through clinical interviews and observations, reviews of other assessment information, and file information. The quality of the judgments they yield depends, then, on the quality of that information and the accuracy with which it is processed. Many of the instruments are designed for use with frontline workers, and this is a strength. However, efforts must always be made to ensure that these workers have the training and supports to conduct the assessments effectively.

Chapter 8

□

Conclusions and Recommendations

The primary objective of this volume was to demonstrate that standardized psychological assessments have an important role to play in the processing of the young offender. More specifically, we were interested in showing that these assessments can enhance the quality of forensic decisions by improving the validity of inferences made about the youth and by encouraging the consistent application of decision rules. We elaborate on these positive contributions of the assessments in the next section.

1. □ Positive Contributions of the Assessments

In Chapter 3, we outlined various potential contributions of standardized psychological assessments to decision making in juvenile justice settings; we are now in a position to illustrate those contributions.

1.1. □ Availability of Tools

Although our review of assessment instruments was not designed to be comprehensive, it still illustrates the large pool of sophisticated tests, rating scales, interview schedules, and other types of instruments and procedures available for assessing the youthful offender. Some of these tools were developed outside the field of forensic psychology, while others have been specifically developed for assessing dimensions relevant to decisions about young offenders. In any case, there are now standardized psychological assessment tools available for virtually all areas of judgment involved in the juvenile justice system.

We have also seen that there are limits to the reliability and validity of these instruments. We will pursue those limits in more detail in a later section of this chapter but will note here some responses to the point. We observe, first, that while there are often limits to the psychometric properties of psychological assessment tools, the inferences yielded by them often represent considerable improvements over the inferences yielded by the casual and unsystematic assessments often conducted in criminal justice settings. This is illustrated, for example, by demonstrations that, while predictions from standardized risk instruments are less than perfect, the level of accuracy often exceeds that based on clinical judgments (Andrews & Bonta, 1994; Clements, 1996). Our second point is that, while there may be limits to the psychometric soundness of the standardized instruments, at least those limits are known; this is in contrast to the situation with unstandardized types of assessments, which have generally not been evaluated. Finally, it is encouraging to note that forensic assessment constitutes an active area of research today, and this research is leading to improvements in existing instruments and the development of new tools.

1.2. □ Consistency

A second potential strength of standardized assessments relates to their role in helping to ensure consistency in assessments and decision making. We saw earlier that anecdotal and empirical evidence exists to support the point that, within many juvenile justice systems, ad hoc and informal procedures are generally followed in assessing the offender, and this frequently leads to variability and inequities in the processing of the youth and what Gottfredson and Gottfredson (1988) refer to as irrational decisions.

Our argument is that the adoption of a standard set of assessment instruments across a system can help to ensure a measure of consistency in assessment and decision making. For example, if all diagnoses of learning disability are based on assessments provided through the WISC-III (Wechsler, 1991), then we have some assurance that the designation "learning disabled" has a consistent meaning. We may also contrast the case where probation officers within a system are given no guidelines in determining risk for future offending with the situation in which all officers employ a standardized tool such as the YLS/CMI (Hoge & Andrews, 1994). Again, we are provided with some insurance that clients are being dealt with in an equitable fashion. The latter type of instrument is particularly important because it is representative of recent efforts to develop assessment tools that systematize forensic judgments. Other examples we saw involve tools for assessing aggravating/mitigating factors and competency to stand trial.

1.3. □ Explicitness of Constructs

A third advantage of using standardized psychological assessments relates to the fact that the constructs represented in the measures are explicit. Admittedly, there are sometimes ambiguities and controversies associated with the theoretical meaning of the constructs, but in most cases there is an operational definition represented in the measure that may be used as a point of reference.

An example of this point may be found with standardized intelligence tests. While there remains controversy over the meaning of the construct of intelligence, standardized intelligence tests represent an explicit set of operational procedures. Furthermore, we now have considerable empirical information about the implications of intelligence test scores for performance in a wide variety of contexts. Another example involves scores from behavioral checklists such as the RBPS (Quay & Peterson, 1987). These instruments yield scores reflecting behavioral dimensions with labels such as anxiety–withdrawal and socialized aggression. These constructs are defined within the measures in terms of specific overt behaviors. Moreover, the considerable research being conducted with these instruments is providing us with information about the implications of these constructs for performance and behavior in different settings.

The use of assessment procedures with explicit operational referents is extremely important from the point of view of explaining and defending our assessments and decisions. Contrast the case where a judgment that a youth is "out of control" is based on a clinical impression from on a one-hour interview with the situation where the judgment is based on a standardized interview yielding a diagnosis that is defined in terms of specific *DSM-IV* criteria. Similarly, a recommendation that a youth be remanded to custody because he or she is extremely high risk for the commission of a violent crime would be more defensible if based on a standardized risk assessment instrument with concrete criteria than if based on appeals to "experience."

1.4. □ Access to Substantive Findings

A fourth argument we put forward in favor of structured psychological assessments relates to Grisso's (1987) call for increased efforts to translate knowledge from other areas of psychology into forensically meaningful terms. We argued that many instruments developed in the fields of educational, social, personality, developmental, and industrial psychology have relevance for the juvenile justice setting and, further, represent means for adapting knowledge developed in those areas to juvenile justice issues.

Two examples in support of the argument are offered. We note, first, that considerable progress is being made in the analysis of the causes, developmental course, and treatment of pathological behaviors in children and adolescents (see, e.g., Kazdin, 1989; Loeber & Stouthamer-Loeber, 1996). Behavioral rating scales and checklists such as the Revised Behavior Problem Checklist and Child Behavior Checklist represent a means of incorporating those developments into decision making regarding the offender.

Our second example relates to the issue of family dynamics. The role of family factors and parenting in delinquency is being actively explored and is yielding important results, as reviews by Henggeler (1989) and Patterson, De-Baryshe, and Ramsey (1989) indicate. Assessment instruments such as the Family Events Checklist (Patterson et al., 1992) and the Weinberger Parenting Inventory

(Feldman & Weinberger, 1994) are designed to reflect this knowledge and represent a means of incorporating the findings into forensic assessments.

1.5. ☐ Evaluation Methodology

Our fifth argument in favor of the use of psychological assessments was based on the fact that the field provides a sophisticated methodology for evaluating the quality of assessments. While there is always some controversy about the integrity of the reliability and validity constructs and the procedures used for assessing them, they are still generally recognized as valuable means of evaluating assessment tools.

We have also seen that limits exist on the adequacy with which the reliability and validity of most of the assessment instruments reviewed has been established. Our main point here, however, is that procedures are available for making the evaluation, and this constitutes an important advantage over the informal and unsystematic assessment procedures generally employed in juvenile justice settings. Assessments of reliability and validity require the use of a standardized format, and most of the informal assessments do not satisfy this criterion.

1.6. ☐ System Efficiency

The arguments we have advanced thus far largely focus on the contributions of psychological assessments to the quality of judgments and decisions made about the youth. We would also like to point out that improvements in this respect have broader implications for juvenile justice systems. Mistakes in decisions can be very costly to the individual offender, the agency, and society. Incarcerations of youths, remands to adult court, and provisions of treatment are all courses of action with very high monetary and human costs, and those costs are often compounded when they represent inappropriate decisions. Wiebush et al. (1995) discuss several empirical demonstrations of this point based on current evaluation research. Similarly, decisions not to incarcerate a youth or not to provide treatment may also be costly when those courses of action are actually justified by circumstances. On a more immediate level, the allocation of resources within a system can be done more efficiently if it is based on an accurate picture of the needs of clients within the system. Structured psychological assessments are capable of providing this information.

2. ☐ Recommendations for Practitioners

The following set of recommendations are relevant to the utilization of psychological assessments in juvenile justice settings. Many of these respond to problems or limitations associated with psychological assessments, which were discussed in Chapter 3 and in the reviews of other chapters.

2.1. □ The Role of Professional Expertise

We can identify several areas of expertise critical to conducting psychological assessments in juvenile justice systems. First, a certain amount of specialized knowledge is required for administering, scoring, and interpreting the measures. The degree of expertise required varies rather widely. At one extreme are those attitudinal rating scales and behavioral checklists that are simple to administer and interpret and require no specialized knowledge. Other measures, such as the YLS/CMI (Hoge & Andrews, 1994), are designed for use by probation officers or other such professionals with special training. Many of the measures, however, call for a higher level of knowledge and experience. The WISC-III and the Psychopathy Checklist (Hare, 1991) are examples. There are detailed training programs associated with these measures, and anyone using the measures should have completed those programs. General criteria regarding the level of qualifications required for different types of measures are set out in the *Standards for Educational and Psychological Testing* (American Psychological Association, 1985).

Note should also be made of computer-aided scoring and interpretation protocols. We are seeing a great increase in the availability of computer-based procedures that will translate raw scores into standardized scores and, in some cases, complete psychological interpretations. Some of these systems are based on empirical analyses and some on clinical judgments. While this type of procedure can be of great assistance to the assessor, it also presents some potential dangers, as Lanyon (1984) and Matarazzo (1986) have observed. The greatest danger is that the availability of these services will encourage use of the measures by individuals without the background to understand the proper use of the assessments.

This relates to the second area of expertise we wish to identify. Not only should the practitioner be expert in the administration and interpretation of the assessment instruments, but it is also important for him or her to have a thorough general background in the area of psychological assessment. We have seen that limits exist with the psychometric properties of all of our instruments and procedures, and it is important that the assessor know those limits and their implications for the judgments and decisions to be made about the client. Related to this is a need for a familiarity with the various ethical guidelines that exist regarding psychological assessments. The major reference in this respect, as we have seen, is the *Standards for Educational and Psychological Testing* of the American Psychological Association (1985), but various state and provincial professional associations may also have guidelines regarding the matter.

A third area of expertise involves a knowledge of the juvenile justice system, including relevant laws, statutes, and policies, and also the administrative structure of the system. A mental health professional cannot function effectively without this knowledge. Among other things, the knowledge is essential from the point of view of communicating with other personnel within the legal system. An important part of the mental health professional's task entails translating the psychological knowledge into terms understandable to judges, lawyers, probation officers, and other such groups. The ability to do that involves a thorough knowledge of the legal system.

A fourth area of expertise relates to an awareness of the literature on the psychology of criminal conduct. We have attempted to show at various points in this book that an impressive body of theoretical and empirical knowledge is being developed regarding the causes of youthful criminal activity and the most effective ways of dealing with that activity. Practitioners are strongly advised to remain current with respect to that literature.

A final area of expertise relates to knowledge and experience in the assessment of children and adolescents. Rogers and Mitchell (1991) make this point in their discussion of evaluations of youthful offenders: "We have steadfastly held to the position that these evaluations should not be done by forensic clinicians who specialize in the assessment and treatment of adults. Developmental issues of late childhood and adolescence cannot be simply translated into adult terms" (p. 293). We have tried to reflect this point in the book by focusing on instruments developed specifically for this age group, but we would also stress that the actual conduct of assessments of young people impose different demands than those with adults.

2.2. ☐ Selection of Instruments

A second set of recommendations concerns the selection of instruments and procedures for use in the system. We have several types of guidelines to offer in this respect.

We note, first, that the selection of assessment tools should be guided by the specific needs of the system. This is the issue of relevance that we raised at the beginning of the volume. The determination of system needs should, in turn, be guided by the objectives of the system and the assumptions made about the best means of achieving those objectives. If, for example, the goal in a particular situation is to reduce the likelihood that a youth will reoffend, and the assumption is made that the best way of achieving that goal is to expose the youth to a period of incarceration consistent with the severity of his or her crime, then the assessment of severity should be the focus of the assessment. If, on the other hand, the assumption is made that the best way of achieving that particular goal is by ameliorating conditions in the youth's environment that are contributing to his or her delinquency, then these environmental factors would constitute the main assessment concerns.

We have seen, however, two general problems that arise in this connection.

First, it is often a challenge to match psychological assessment tools with legal constructs. There is often a considerable discrepancy between legal and psychological constructs, even where the terminology sounds similar. Amenability to treatment is one of many examples of the point, which we discussed earlier.

The second problem is that in many juvenile justice systems there is a lack of clarity and consistency regarding goals and guiding assumptions and even the meaning of the legal constructs. There are, to be sure, continuing efforts to refine the legal constructs and to develop concrete "decision standards," but it is widely recognized that considerable uncertainty still exists within legal systems (see, e.g., Grisso, 1987; Grisso et al., 1988; Melton et al., 1987). This situation is often beyond the control of the mental health provider responsible for assessments, but it is important to recognize that the ability to make intelligent selections of assessment tools is limited when this clarity is absent.

It is also important to recognize that enhanced clarity within the system may help address some of the other potential dangers of psychological assessments discussed in Chapter 3. We saw there the criticism that the use of psychological assessments has sometimes encouraged too much of a focus on individual characteristics and too little concern with the environmental characteristics of the youth. Where the objectives and operating policies of the system have been thoroughly worked out, however, the entire range of variables thought relevant to the system will become clear. A similar point may be made in connection with the objection that the use of psychological assessments will result in a "widening of the net." This situation will not occur in systems in which concrete and explicit guidelines exist with respect to the behaviors and activities that fall within the scope of the system. In these cases, the treatment of youths will not be dictated by the assessment instruments employed but by the policies of the system.

Having established what the needs of the system are, the next task is to select the best available instruments and procedures for addressing the concerns. This depends on the mental health provider responsible for the assessments being aware of the latest developments in the field. This should involve more than a perusal of the latest test publisher catalogues (not always the best source of information about the measures) and should include exposure to journals and basic reference tools such as the *Mental Measurements Yearbook* (Conoley & Impara, 1995) and *Test Critiques* (Keyser & Sweetland, 1992). Progress in the field of assessment is rapid, and it is important to be current regarding new developments. Also important is an awareness of professionals in the community capable of providing specialized assessments that may be beyond the capacities of the assessor. Included would be specialists in neuropsychological, learning disability, and career assessments.

Formation of assessment batteries also constitutes an important part of the planning process. There are situations in which the assessment needs are relatively specific—e.g., the assessor is asked to provide information about cognitive functioning or about social competencies. In most cases, however, a broader assessment is called for. For example, predisposition assessments usually call for information about a broad range of dimensions, including the youth's family situation, peer group associations, cognitive functioning, personality traits, and behavioral dispositions. Similarly, judgments of mental competency for use in waiver and transfer decisions generally require information about a set of factors. Both of these situations require groups or batteries of assessment instruments.

There are several rules to be observed in forming these batteries. First, the batteries should include measuring devices assessing the full range of variables relevant to the decision. Second, where possible, multiple sources of information should be employed. Information about the youth's circumstances and characteristics collected independently from the youth, his or her parents, teachers, police, and childcare workers with prior experience with the child can be very useful. Achenbach's efforts to develop parallel instruments for a variety of sources (youth, parent, teacher) and in a variety of formats (checklists, observation schedules, interview schedules) may be an important resource in this respect (see Achenbach & McConaughy, 1987). Third, the instruments should be organized in such a way so as to bear logically on the decision to be made.

One useful model of an assessment battery for use in juvenile justice systems is that presented by Jaffe et al. (1985). The model entails four stages. The first of these is designed to provide a social history and a thorough assessment of the personality and behavioral characteristics of the youth and includes a social history interview and a set of standardized personality tests. The latter includes the Basic Personality Inventory (Jackson, 1995) and Bennett's Self-Esteem Scale (Bennett, Sorensen, & Forshag, 1971). Stage II represents an effort to explore problem areas identified in Stage I more intensively through interviews and file information. Stage III then involves an integration of information collected in the first two stages, while the final stage involves an implementation of the case plan developed in Stage III. The authors describe the application of this model in a family court clinic.

We have outlined in Figure 8.1 an example of another intake assessment battery. This battery would be appropriate when an intensive assessment of an older offender (age 15–17) is required. It includes measures encompassing a broad range of risk, need, and responsivity factors. Where necessary, additional data could also be solicited from other professionals (police, probation officers) or from file information. The YLS/CMI is suggested as a means of summarizing the information collected in the battery and of formulating a case plan based on the assessment.

Several other efforts to develop composite assessments also bear mention. Wormith (1995) has developed a system for assessing risk and need levels appropriate for older young offenders (16- and 17-year-olds). The system involves, first, a checklist instrument similar to the YLS/CMI. This provides an initial estimate of

Structured interview
Revised Diagnostic Interview Schedule for Children and Adolescents (Shaffer et al., 1993)

Aptitude measure
Multidimensional Aptitude Battery (Research Psychologists Press/Sigma)

Personality tests
Basic Personality Inventory (Research Psychologists Press/Sigma)
Multidimensional Self-Concept Scale (PRO-ED)

Attitudinal measures
Criminal Sentiments Scale (Gendreau et al., 1979)
Pride in Delinquency Scale (Shields & Whitehall, 1991)

Measure of behavioral pathology–parent
Child Behavior Checklist (University Associates in Psychiatry)

Measure of behavioral pathology and school performance–teacher
Child Behavior Checklist–Teacher Report Form (University Associates in Psychiatry)

Broad-based risk/need assessment
Youth Level of Service/Case Management Inventory (Hoge & Andrews, 1994)

Figure 8.1. □ Model intake assessment battery.

risk and need levels. Risk and need areas identified in this first phase are then explored through more thorough assessments conducted on the basis of specific assessment protocols.

Another type of model is one developed for screening youths at risk for delinquency and conduct disorders. This is primarily designed to identify youths before they become delinquent, but it also has some application for judging risk and need levels of adjudicated offenders. The model involves a multiple gating procedure in which relatively nonintrusive assessments are conducted for initial screening and more intensive assessments are introduced as clients "pass" succeeding gates. The major advantage of this type of model is that it reserves the more intrusive (and expensive) assessments for those identified as higher risk. Both August, Realmuto, Crosby, and MacDonald (1995) and Loeber, Dishion, & Patterson (1984) have presented examples of this type of model.

3. □ Research Recommendations

In this section, we identify a number of areas relevant to psychological assessments in which there are important research needs.

3.1. ☐ Criminological Processes

The primary route to improved psychological assessments is through advances in our understanding of antisocial behavior in youth. As we develop a better comprehension of the factors that cause delinquent and other antisocial behaviors and of the way in which youths react to different interventions and treatments, we will be in a position to develop more valid and more relevant assessment tools.

There are a variety of very active areas of theory and research that are providing important directions in this respect. As we have seen, there are numerous efforts to develop theoretical models of criminal activity that integrate a wide range of causal variables (e.g., Andrews & Bonta, 1994; Andrews et al., 1990; Elliott et al., 1985; Hawkins et al., 1995; Le Blanc et al., 1988). Associated with these models is a growing body of empirical research on the causes of youth crime, the developmental course of antisocial behaviors, and criminal typologies. Significant progress is being made in this research as revealed in recent reviews by Andrews and Bonta (1994); Andrews et al. (1992); Henggeler (1989, 1991); Loeber & Stouthamer-Loeber (1987, 1996); Thornberry, Huizinga, and Loeber (1995); and Yoshikawa (1995).

Parallel to the work focusing specifically on young offenders are theoretical and empirical efforts in child and adolescent psychology directed toward the analysis of the developmental processes associated with a wide range of pathological behaviors. Reviews of this research by Hawkins, Catalano, and Miller (1992); Hersen and Ammerman (1995); Kazdin (1987, 1989); and Tremblay (1992) reveal that here, too, considerable progress is being made in understanding the developmental processes involved in the origin and evolution of antisocial behaviors.

This basic work within criminology, psychology, and other social science areas is relevant to the assessment of the full range of judgmental areas discussed in this volume. For example, our ability to assess risk for future violent activity rests very directly on an understanding of the factors that contribute to this activity. Advances in our basic knowledge about youthful criminal activity will also lead to improvements in our ability to assess aggravating and mitigating factors, mental competency, criminogenic needs, and responsivity to treatment.

Program evaluation research on the effectiveness of different types of interventions for youthful offenders is also important in the development of improved assessment tools. Reviews by Andrews and Bonta (1994); Andrews et al. (1990); Lipsey and Wilson (1993); Mulvey, Arthur, and Reppucci (1993); Palmer (1994); and Tate, Reppucci, and Mulvey (1995) reveal that the debate over the effectiveness of various interventions for delinquent youth (including punitive sanctions and various treatment approaches) remains a subject of considerable debate. On the other hand, as Andrews and Bonta (1994) and Andrews et al. (1990) have argued, there is emerging support for the position that there are effective interventions for delinquent youth. Their analysis also makes clear, however, that these interventions are effective to the extent that they are matched with the specific need and responsivity characteristics of the youth and are delivered effectively. This conclusion is based at present on a small but growing empirical base.

Kazdin's (1987, 1993) reviews of research on the treatment of disturbed youth from the more general area of child and adolescent psychology also appear to support the conclusion that there are effective interventions for childhood disorders. Especially encouraging, too, is the growing evidence that some early intervention programs can be effective in protecting youths from factors contributing to criminal activity. Reviews of this work have been presented by Hawkins and Catalano (1992), Hawkins et al., (1995), and Yoshikawa (1994).

This research on the effectiveness of various interventions for young offenders is very important from the point of view of selecting and developing assessment tools. Decisions about dispositions, levels of security, placement in programs, and referrals for treatment all depend on judgments about amenability to treatment, risk levels, criminogenic needs, and responsivity factors. Those judgments, in turn, are guided by the assumptions we make about the relative effectiveness of different types of interventions for different types of youths, and the validity of those assumptions depends very directly on an accurate understanding of the dynamics of the intervention process. For example, our ability to choose aptitude and personality tests to select youths who will benefit from a particular intervention program depends directly on our understanding of the dynamics of that particular program.

3.2. □ Construct Development

Another area needing research attention relates to the definition of constructs. It should be clear that all of the psychological assessment tools entail constructs of some sort, and those constructs are important because they guide the judgments and decisions that follow from the assessments. For example, the Basic Personality Inventory (Jackson, 1995) described earlier is scored in terms of constructs such as depression, alienation, and social introversion. Other constructs yielded by the various types of measures include conduct disorder, borderline retarded, anxious, high risk, etc. Decisions about the youth are then based on scores from these dimensions.

We had earlier made the argument that standardized psychological assessments have an advantage over less standardized types of assessments because they generally offer an explicit operational definition of constructs. This is true, but it must be acknowledged that there sometimes exist ambiguities about the actual meaning of constructs (see, e.g., Quay et al., 1987; Waldman et al., 1995). The efforts of Hoge and Andrews (1992) and Loeber, Keenan, Lahey, Green, and Thomas (1993) to analyze and clarify the conduct disorder construct is illustrative of the type of effort needed in this area.

The meaningfulness of the constructs represented in our psychological measures constitutes one area of concern. A second area of concern relates to the meaningfulness of the legal constructs represented in the juvenile justice system. We are referring to constructs such as amenability to treatment, competency to stand trial, aggravating factors, and others. These constructs are, in a sense, beyond the scope of psychological research. Definitions of legal constructs rest with the judicial and legislative systems. It has been suggested, however, that social science research can contribute to an explication of the constructs:

> The problem suggests the need for *systematic inquiry into the conceptual and empirical relations between (a) information about juveniles and (b) legal standards controlling juvenile court decisions.* It is beyond the scope of social science research, of course, to determine what types of information satisfy the law's ultimate purpose. Yet where the law is vague in its guidance to legal decision makers in the use of information, social science methods can assist the law by examining the range of information available for decisions, structuring the diversity of information, and examining courts' current uses of information in relation to legal decisions. (Grisso et al., 1988, p. 404; italics in original)

This work is also important from the point of view of clarifying the relation between the constructs represented in psychological assessments and the legal judgments they are designed to inform.

Grisso et al.'s (1988) research on the psychosocial correlates of decisions regarding detention, transfers, and postdisposition choice is representative of the work required in this area. Another good example of this type of effort is Roesch's (Roesch & Golding, 1987; Roesch, Ogloff, & Golding, 1993) efforts to clarify the construct of competency to stand trial. Part of this approach has involved an effort to analyze the relation between the legal construct of competency and the kind of information conveyed in standardized instruments for assessing competency.

3.3. ☐ Instrument Development

A third critical area of research concerns the development, evaluation, and refinement of instruments and procedures for assessing the youthful offender. Several directions for research may be identified.

First, there is a continuing need to identify and adapt to the judicial setting instruments developed in child, social, personality, educational and other areas of psychology. As we have tried to show, there are exciting assessment developments in those areas, and many of those have relevance for the juvenile justice setting. It is also important, however, to ensure that the instruments are relevant to the judgments and decisions called for in that setting (Grisso, 1987). Efforts should focus, therefore, on the establishment of norms applicable to young offenders and assessments of the reliability and validity of the instruments with specific reference to forensic decisions. It is important, for example, to be able to demonstrate that tests and rating instruments exhibit what we referred to as treatment validity, that is, the capacity to meaningfully track changes in the client resulting from intervention efforts.

Examples of efforts to adapt existing assessment instruments to the justice setting may be found in earlier work with the MMPI (Zager, 1988) and in the more recent efforts to relate the BPI to the assessment of adolescent offenders (e.g., Leschied et al., 1988).

The second line of research involves developing and evaluating instruments specifically for the justice system. The need for such research was argued by Grisso (1987), and there has been considerable response to that call at the adult level. There has been somewhat less research activity in the development of forensic instruments applicable to children and adults, but there is growing interest in the issue. This is illustrated, as we saw, in recent efforts to develop typology/classification systems and risk instruments specifically for youthful offenders. Related to this are calls for more attention to the special assessment needs of young offenders from specific cultural groups (e.g., Hammond & Yung, 1993; Reitsma-Street, 1991) and of different offender groups, such as sex offenders (e.g., Knight & Prenky, 1993). In sum, there remain many challenges for researchers interested in the development of forensic assessment tools.

4. □ Concluding Comments

Our primary goal in this volume has been to show how standardized psychological assessments can contribute to a more effective management of youth within juvenile justice systems. We have addressed issues regarding the treatment of youthful offenders only as they have had a bearing on the assessment issue. We would like to conclude, however, with a few final comments on the treatment of youth crime.

There are vigorous controversies over the extent of youth crime and the most appropriate way of dealing with the problem; there is less debate over the high costs associated with youthful criminal activity. These costs relate to the financial and emotional harm suffered by victims of the crime and, in many cases, the offender and his or her family. In addition, there are the significant monetary costs associated with maintaining the law enforcement and judicial systems created for dealing with the criminal activity. In the longer term, there are the tremendous financial and social costs associated with failures to deal effectively with the problem of criminal activity during childhood or adolescence; we are referring to the case in which this failure is then associated with adult antisocial behavior. Finally, one other area of "cost" should also be assessed: those costs incurred when a fear of youth crime leads us to actions that are inconsistent with fundamental democratic ideals regarding equity, fairness, and humane treatment.

We indicated at the beginning of the book that we favor a child welfare or rehabilitative approach to the problem of youth crime. We feel that the treatment of the youthful offender should begin by identifying the specific criminogenic needs of the youth, that is, the factors that are directly associated with his or her criminal activity. Those needs should then be addressed through the delivery of programs (preferably community-based) that are (1) matched to the criminogenic needs and responsivity characteristics of the youth; (2) proven effective for the problem in question; and (3) delivered effectively.

However, whatever position is favored regarding the treatment of youth crime, the high social and financial costs associated with this activity make it absolutely imperative that we recognize this as an issue of paramount concern and adopt a willingness to commit whatever resources are needed to address the problem. The potential profits from this commitment are immense.

Appendix 1 □

Instruments and Procedures Identified in This Volume

The source or reference for each instrument/procedure follows it in parentheses.

Chapter 4

Armed Services Vocational Aptitude Battery (United States Department of Defense)

Bennett Mechanical Comprehension Test (The Psychological Corporation)

Career Assessment Inventory (Interpretive Scoring Systems)

Classroom Reading Inventory (Wm. C. Brown)

Cognitive Abilities Test (Houghton-Mifflin)

Detroit Tests of Learning Aptitudes (PRO-ED)

Differential Aptitude Test (The Psychological Corporation)

Goodenough-Harris Drawing Test (The Psychological Corporation)

Halstead-Reitan Neuropsychological Test Battery for Older Children (Neuropsychology Press)

Henmon-Nelson Test (Houghton-Mifflin)

Illinois Test of Psycholinguistic Abilities (University of Illinois Press)

Jackson Vocational Interest Survey (Research Psychologists Press/Sigma)

Kaufman Assessment Battery for Children (American Guidance Service)

Kaufman Test of Educational Achievement (American Guidance Service)

Keymath Diagnostic Arithmetic Test (American Guidance Service)

Kuhlmann-Anderson Test (Personnel Press)

Leiter International Performance Scale (C.H. Stoelting Co.)

Multidimensional Aptitude Battery (Research Psychologists Press/Sigma)

Occupational Aptitude Survey and Interest Schedule (PRO-ED)

Peabody Individual Achievement Test–Revised (American Guidance Service)

Peabody Picture Vocabulary Test (American Guidance Service)

Quick Neurological Screening Test–Revised (Psychological Corporation)

Raven's Progressive Matrices (Lewis Publishing Co.)

Self-Directed Search Inventory (Psychological Assessment Resources)

Shipley Institute of Living Scale (Western Psychological Services)

Stanford Achievement Test (Psychological Corporation)

Stanford-Binet Intelligence Scale (4th ed.) (Houghton-Mifflin)
Strong-Campbell Interest Inventory (Consulting Psychologists Press)
Test of Auditory Comprehension of Language (DLM Teaching Resources)
Wechsler Adult Intelligence Scale–Revised (The Psychological Corporation)
Wechsler Intelligence Scale for Children III (The Psychological Corporation)
Wide Range Achievement Test–Revised (The Psychological Corporation)
Woodcock-Johnson Psycho-Educational Battery (DLM Teaching Resources)

Chapter 5

AAMD Adaptive Behavior Scale-School Edition (PRO-ED)
Adaptive Behavior Evaluation Scale (Hawthorne Educational Services)
Adjustment Scale for Children and Adolescents (McDermott, Marston, & Stott, 1993)
Adolescent Drinking Index (Research Psychologists Press/Sigma)
Adolescent Drug Abuse Diagnostic Instrument (Friedman & Utada, 1989)
Adolescent Problem Inventory (Freedman et al., 1978)
Antisocial Behaviours Scale (Forth & Brown, 1993)
Attitudes Toward Institutional Authority (Rigby, 1982)
Attitudes Toward Legal Agencies (Shaw & Wright, 1967)
Attitudes Toward Probation Officers (Shaw & Wright, 1967)
Basic Personality Inventory (Research Psychologists Press/Sigma)
Behavior Assessment System for Children (Reynolds & Kamphaus, 1992)
Brief Psychiatric Rating Scale for Children (Overall & Pfefferbaum, 1982)
Child Assessment Schedule (Hodges, 1985)
Child Behavior Checklist (Parent) (University Associates in Psychiatry/Guidance Centre)
Classroom Observation Code (Abikoff & Gittelman, 1985)
Child Behavior Checklist (Teacher) (University Associates in Psychiatry/ Guidance Centre)
Conners Teacher Rating Scale (Multi-Health Systems)
Criminal Sentiments Scale (Gendreau et al., 1979)
Culture-Free Self-Esteem Inventory (Research Psychologists Press)
Devereux Adolescent Behavior Rating Scale (Devereux Foundation)
Diagnostic Interview Schedule for Children (Costello et al., 1984)
Diagnostic Interview for Children and Adolescents (Herjanic et al., 1975)
Direct Observation Form (University Associates in Psychiatry)
Drug Abuse Screening Test (Skinner, 1982)
Drug Use Screening Inventory (Tarter, 1990)
Eating Disorder Inventory–2 (Garner, 1996)
High School Personality Questionnaire (The Psychological Corporation)
Independent Living Behavior Checklist (West Virginia Research and Training Center)

Interview for Antisocial Behavior (Kazdin & Esveldt-Dawson, 1986)
Jesness Inventory (Consulting Psychologists Press)
Millon Adolescent Personality Inventory (National Computer Systems)
Minnesota Multiphasic Personality Inventory (National Computer Systems)
Multidimensional Self-Concept Scale (PRO-ED)
Neutralization Scale (Shields & Whitehall, 1994)
Normative Adaptive Behavior Checklist (The Psychological Corporation)
Personality Inventory for Youth (Western Psychological Services)
Piers-Harris Children's Self-Concept Scale (Western Psychological Services)
Pride in Delinquency Scale (Shields & Whitehall, 1991)
Psychopathy Checklist (Hare, 1991)
Revised Behavior Problem Checklist (Quay & Peterson, 1987)
Revised Diagnostic Interview Schedule for Children and Adolescents (Shaffer et al., 1993)
Revised Legal Attitudes Questionnaire (Kravitz et al., 1993)
Reynolds Adolescent Depression Scale (Psychological Assessment Resources)
Scales of Independent Behavior (Bruininks et al., 1984)
Self-Description Questionnaire (Marsh & O'Neill, 1984)
Self-Esteem Index (Psychological Assessment Resources)
Self-Report Deliquency Scale (Elliott et al., 1989)
Self-Reported Delinquency Scale (Mak, 1993)
Semistructured Clinical Interview for Children (McConaughy & Achenbach, 1990)
Suicidal Ideation Questionnaire (Research Psychologists Press/Sigma)
Vineland Adaptive Behavior Scales (Sparrow et al., 1984)
Youth Self-Report Inventory (University Associates in Psychiatry/Guidance Centre)

Chapter 6

Children's Report of Parental Behavior Inventory (Schluderman & Schluderman, 1970)
Community-Oriented Environment Program Scale (Moos, 1986b)
Correctional Institutions Environment Scale (Moos, 1986a)
Correctional Program Assessment Inventory (Gendreau & Andrews, 1994)
Family Adaptability and Cohesion Evaluation (Olson et al., 1985)
Family Assessment Device (Epstein et al., 1983)
Family Assessment Measure III (Multi-Health Systems)
Family Beliefs Inventory (Roehling & Robin, 1986)
Family Environment Scale (Moos & Moos, 1986)
Family Events Checklist (Patterson et al., 1992)
Parent–Adolescent Relationship Questionnaire (Robin et al., 1990)
Parent Practices Scale (Strayhorn & Weidman, 1988)
Parenting Risk Scale (Mrazek et al., 1995)

Prison Environment Inventory (Wright, 1985)
Weinberger Parenting Inventory (Feldman & Weinberger, 1994)

Chapter 7

Arizona Juvenile Risk Assessment Form (Ashford et al., 1986)
Competence Assessment for Standing Trial for Defendants with Mental Retardation (Everington & Dunn, 1995)
Competency to Stand Trial Assessment Instrument (Weisstub, 1984)
Conceptual Level Matching Model (CLMM) (Reitsma-Street & Leschied, 1988)
Diagnostic and Statistical Manual of Mental Disorders (4th ed.) (DSM-IV) (American Psychiatric Association, 1994)
Firesetting Risk Interview (Kolko & Kazdin, 1989)
Fitness Interview Test (Roesch et al., 1984)
Interpersonal Maturity Level Classification System (I-Level) (Warren, 1983)
Minnesota Multiphasic Personality Inventory (MMPI) (National Computer Systems)
Psychopathy Checklist–Revised (Multi-Health Systems)
Sentencing Factors Inventory (Andrews et al., 1987)
Wisconsin Juvenile Probation and Aftercare Assessment Form (Baird, 1981, 1985)
Youth Level of Service/Case Management Inventory (Hoge & Andrews, 1994)

Appendix 2

⌐

Addresses of Major Test Publishers

American Guidance Service, P. O. Box 99, Circle Pines, MN 55014-1796
C. H. Stoelting Co., 620 Wheat Lane, Wood Dale, IL 60191
Consulting Psychologists Press, P. O. Box 10096, Palo Alto, CA 94303
CTB/Macmillan/McGraw-Hill, 2500 Garden Rd., Monterey, CA 93940
Devereux Foundation, 19 S. Waterloo Rd., P. O. Box 400, Devon, PA 19333
DLM Teaching Resources, One DLM Park, Allen, TX 75002
Grune & Stratton, 465 South Lincoln Dr., Troy, MO 63379
Guidance Centre, 712 Gordon Baker Rd., Toronto, Ontario M2H 3R7
Hawthorne Educational Services, 800 Gray Oak Dr., Columbia, MO 65201
Houghton-Mifflin, 222 Berkeley St., Boston, MA 02116
Interpretive Scoring Systems, 4401 West 76th St., Minneapolis, MN 55435
Jastak Associates, Inc., P. O. Box 3410, Wilmington, DE 19804
Lewis Publishing Co., 136 Gower St., London WCIE 6BS, United Kingdom
Multi-Health Systems, 908 Niagara Falls Blvd., North Tonawanda, NY 14120-2060
Multi-Health Systems (Canada), 5 Overlea Blvd., Suite 210, Toronto, Ontario M4H 1P1
National Computer Systems, P. O. Box 1416, Minneapolis, MN 55440
Personnel Press, 191 Spring St., Lexington, MA 02173
PRO-ED, 8700 Shoal Creek Blvd., Austin, TX 78757
Psychological Assessment Resources, P. O. Box 998, Odessa, FL 33556
The Psychological Corporation, P. O. Box 839954, San Antonio, TX 78283-3954
The Psychological Corporation (Canada), 55 Horner Ave., Toronto, Ontario M8Z 4X6
Reitan Neuropsychology Laboratories, 2920 South 4th Ave., Tucson, AZ 85713-4819
Research Psychologists Press, P. O. Box 3292, Station B, London, Ontario N6A 4K3
Sigma Assessment Systems, P. O. Box 610984, Port Huron, MI 48061
Slosson Educational Publications, P. O. Box 280, East Aurora, NY 14052
United States Department of Defense, Testing Directorate, 2500 Green Bay Rd., North Chicago, IL 60064

University Associates in Psychiatry, Department of Psychiatry, University of Vermont, Burlington, VT 05401

University of Illinois Press, 54 E. Gregory Dr., Champaign, IL 61820

West Virginia Research and Training Center, 509 Allen Hall, West Virginia University, Morgantown, WV 26506

Western Psychological Services, 12031 Wilshire Blvd., Los Angeles, CA 90025

References

Abikoff, H., & Gittelman, R. (1985). Classroom Observation Code: A modification of the Stony Brook Code. *Psychopharmacology Bulletin, 21,* 901–909.

Achenbach, T. M. (1991a). *Manual for the Child Behavior Checklist/4–18 and 1991 Profile.* Burlington, VT: University of Vermont, Department of Psychiatry.

Achenbach, T. M. (1991b). *Manual for the Teacher's Report Form and 1991 Profile.* Burlington, VT: University of Vermont, Department of Psychiatry.

Achenbach, T. M., & McConaughy, S. H. (1987). *Empirically based assessment of child and adolescent psychopathology: Practical applications.* Newbury Park, CA: Sage.

Akers, R. L. (1994). *Criminological theories: Introduction and evaluation.* Los Angeles, CA: Roxbury.

American Psychiatric Association. (1989). *Principles of medical ethics with annotations especially applicable to psychiatry.* Washington, DC: Author.

American Psychiatric Association. (1994). *Diagnostic and statistical manual of mental disorders* (4th ed.). Washington, DC: Author.

American Psychological Association. (1985). *Standards for educational and psychological testing.* Washington, DC: Author.

American Psychological Association. (1991). *Ethical guidelines for forensic psychology.* Washington, DC: Author.

Anastasi, A. (1986). Evolving concepts of test validation. *Annual Review of Psychology, 37,* 1–15.

Andrews, D. A., & Bonta, J. (1994). *The psychology of criminal conduct.* Cincinnati, OH: Anderson Publishing.

Andrews, D. A., & Bonta, J. (1995). *Level of Service Inventory-Revised.* Toronto: Multi-Health Systems.

Andrews, D. A., Bonta, J., & Hoge, R. D. (1990). Classification for effective rehabilitation: Rediscovering psychology. *Criminal Justice and Behavior, 17,* 19–52.

Andrews, D. A., Hoge, R. D., & Leschied, A. (1992). *A review of the profile, classification, and treatment literature with young offenders: A social psychological analysis.* Toronto: Ontario Ministry of Community and Social Services.

Andrews, D. A., Robblee, M. A., Saunders, R., Huartson, K., Robinson, D., Kiessling, J. J., & West, D. (1987). Some psychometrics of judicial decision-making: Toward a Sentencing Factors Inventory. *Criminal Justice and Behavior, 14,* 62–80.

Andrews, D. A., Robinson, D., & Hoge, R. D. (1984). *Manual for the Youth Level of Service Inventory.* Ottawa, Ontario: Department of Psychology, Carleton University.

Archer, R. P. (1989). *MMPI assessment of adolescent clients: Clinical notes on the MMPI, No. 12.* Minneapolis, MN: National Computer Systems.

Archer, R. P. (1992). *MMPI-A: Assessing adolescent psychopathology.* Hillsdale, NJ: Lawrence Erlbaum Associates.

Ashford, J. B., & LeCroy, C. W. (1988). Predicting recidivism: An evaluation of the Wisconsin Juvenile Probation and Aftercare Risk Instrument. *Criminal Justice and Behavior, 15,* 141–151.

Ashford, J. B., & LeCroy, C. W. (1990). Juvenile recidivism: A comparison of three prediction instruments. *Adolescence, 25,* 441–450.

Ashford, J. B., LeCroy, C. W., & Bond-Maupin, L. (1986). *The Arizona Juvenile Aftercare Decision Making System*. Tempe, AZ: Arizona State University.

August, G. J., Realmuto, G. M., Crosby, R. D., & MacDonald III, A. W. (1995). Community-based multiple-gate screening of children at risk for conduct disorder. *Journal of Abnormal Child Psychology, 23*, 521–544.

Baird, S. C. (1981). Probation and parole classification: The Wisconsin model. *Corrections Today, 43*, 36–41.

Baird, S. C. (1984). *Classification of juveniles in corrections: A model systems approach*. Washington, DC: Arthur D. Little.

Baird, S. C. (1985). Classifying juveniles: Making the most of an important management tool. *Corrections Today, 47*, 32–38.

Bala, N. (1992). The Young Offenders Act: The legal structure. In R. R. Corrado, N. Bala, R. Linden, & M. Le Blanc (Eds.), *Juvenile justice in Canada: A theoretical and analytical assessment* (pp. 21–73). Toronto: Butterworths.

Bennett, L. A., Sorensen, D. E., & Forshag, H. (1971). The application of self-esteem measures in correctional settings: I. Reliability of the scale and relationship to other measures. *Journal of Research in Crime and Deliquency, 8*, 1–9.

Beutler, L. E., & Clarkin, J. (1990). *Systematic treatment selection: Toward targeted therapeutic interventions*. New York: Brunner/Mazel.

Billings, A., & Moos, R. (1982). Family environments and adaptation: A clinically applicable typology. *American Journal of Family Therapy, 10*, 26–38.

Binder, A., Geis, G., & Bruce, D. (1988). *Juvenile delinquency: Historical, cultural, and legal perspectives*. New York: Macmillan.

Blaske, D. M., Borduin, C. M., Henggeler, S. W., & Mann, B. J. (1989). Individual, family, and peer characteristics of adolescent sex offenders and assaultive offenders. *Developmental Psychology, 25*, 846–855.

Borduin, C. M., Mann, B. J., Cone, L. T., Henggeler, S. W., Fucci, B. R., Blaske, D. M., & Williams, R. A. (1995). Multisystemic treatment of serious juvenile offenders: Long-term prevention of criminality and violence. *Journal of Consulting and Clinical Psychology, 63*, 569–578.

Brodsky, S. L., & Smitherman, H. W. (1983). *Handbook of scales for research in crime and delinquency*. New York: Plenum.

Bronfenbrenner, U. (1979). *The ecology of human development*. Cambridge, MA: Harvard University Press.

Bronfenbrenner, U. (1986). Ecology of the family as a context for human development: Research perspectives. *Developmental Psychology, 22*, 723–742.

Bruininks, R. H., Woodcock, R. W., Weatherman, R. F., & Hill, B. K. (1984). *Scales of Independent Behavior: Interviewer's manual*. Allen, TX: DLM Teaching Resources.

Butcher, J. N., Williams, C. L., Graham, J. R., Archer, R. P., Tellegen, R. P., Ben- Porath, Y. S., & Kaemmer, B. (1992). *MMPI-A: Manual for administration, scoring, and interpretation*. Minneapolis, MN: University of Minnesota Press.

Butler, J. W., Novy, D., Kagan, N., & Gates, G. (1994). An investigation of differences in attitudes between suicidal and nonsuicidal student ideators. *Adolescence, 29*, 623–628.

Byrne, B. M. (1984). The general/academic self-concept nomological network: A review of construct validation research. *Review of Educational Research, 54*, 427–456.

Byrne, B. M. (1996). *Measuring self-concept across the life span: Issues and instrumentation*. Washington, DC: American Psychological Association.

Campbell, D. T., & Fiske, D. W. (1959). Convergent and discriminant validation by the multitrait-multimethod matrix. *Psychological Bulletin, 56*, 81–105.

Canadian Psychological Association (1991). *Canadian Code of Ethics for Psychologists*. Ottawa, Ontario: Author.

Canter, M. B., Bennett, B. E., Jones, S. E., & Nagy, T. F. (1994). *Ethics for psychologists: A commentary on the APA Ethics Code.* Washington, DC: American Psychological Association.

Carrington, P. J., Moyer, S., & Kopelman, F. (1988). Factors affecting predispositional detention and release in Canadian juvenile courts. *Journal of Criminal Justice, 16,* 463–476.

Carrow-Woolfolk, E. (1985). *Test for Auditory Comprehension of Language* (Rev. Ed.). Allen, TX: DLM Teaching Resources.

Champion, D. J. (1994). *Measuring offender risk: A criminal justice sourcebook.* Westport, CT: Greenwood Press.

Clear, T. (1988). Statistical prediction in corrections. *Research in Corrections, 1,* 1–39.

Clements, C. B. (1981). The future of offender classification: Some cautions and prospects. *Criminal Justice and Behavior, 8,* 15–35.

Clements, C. B. (1996). Offender classification: Two decades of progress. *Criminal Justice and Behavior, 23,* 121–143.

Cline, T. (1985). Clinical judgment in context: A review of situational factors in person perception during clinical interviews. *Journal of Child Psychology and Psychiatry, 26,* 369–380.

Cohen, S. (1985). *Visions of social control: Crime, punishment, and classification.* Oxford: Basil Blackwell.

Compas, B. E., Hinden, B. R., & Gerhardt, C. A. (1995). Adolescent development: Pathways and processes of risk and resilience. *Annual Review of Psychology, 46,* 265–293.

Conoley, J. C., & Impara, J. C. (1995). *The 12th mental measurements yearbook.* Lincoln, NB: University of Nebraska Press.

Corrado, R. R. (1992). Introduction. In R. R. Corrado, N. Bala, R. Linden, & M. Le Blanc (Eds.), *Juvenile justice in Canada: A theoretical and analytical assessment* (pp. 1–20). Toronto: Butterworths.

Corrado, R. R., & Markwart, A. (1992). The evolution and implementation of a new era in juvenile justice in Canada. In R. R. Corrado, N. Bala, R. Linden, & M. Le Blanc (Eds.), *Juvenile justice in Canada: A theoretical and analytical assessment* (pp. 137–228). Toronto: Butterworths.

Corrado, R. R., & Turnbull, S. D. (1992). A comparative examination of the Modified Justice Model in the United Kingdom and the United States. In R. R. Corrado, N. Bala, R. Linden, & M. Le Blanc (Eds.), *Juvenile justice in Canada: A theoretical and analytical assessment* (pp. 75–136). Toronto: Butterworths.

Costello, E. J., Edelbrock, L. S., Dulcan, M. K., Kalas, R., & Klaric, S. H. (1984). *Report on the NIMH Diagnostic Interview Schedule for Children (DISC).* Washington, DC: National Institute of Mental Health.

Crealock, C. M. (1991). Characteristics and needs of the learning-disabled young offender. In A. W. Leschied, P. G. Jaffe, and W. Willis (Eds.), *The Young Offenders Act: A revolution in Canadian juvenile justice* (pp. 233–247). Toronto: University of Toronto Press.

Dannefer, D., & Shutt, R. (1982). Race and juvenile justice processing in court and police agencies. *American Journal of Sociology, 87,* 1113–1132.

Dawes, R. M., Faust, D., & Meehl, P. E. (1989). Clinical vs actuarial judgments. *Science, 243,* 1668–1674.

Doob, A. N., & Beaulieu, L. A. (1993). Variation in the exercise of judicial discretion with young offenders. In T. O'Reilly-Fleming & B. Clark (Eds.), *Youth injustice: Canadian perspectives* (pp. 231–248). Toronto: Canadian Scholars Press.

Doob, A. N., & Chan, J. B. L. (1982). Factors affecting police decisions to take juveniles to court. *Canadian Journal of Criminology, 24,* 25–37.

Doob, A. N., & Chan, J. B. L. (1993). Trends in the use of custodial dispositions with young offenders. In T. O'Reilly-Fleming & B. Clark (Eds.), *Youth injustice: Canadian perspectives* (pp. 249–276). Toronto: Canadian Scholars Press.

Elliott, D. S., Ageton, S. S., Huizinga, D., Knowles, B. A., & Canter, R. J. (1983). *The prevalence and incidence of delinquent behavior: 1976–1980.* Boulder, CO: Behavioral Research Institute.

Elliott, D. S., Huizinga, D., & Ageton, S. S. (1985). *Explaining delinquency and drug use.* Beverly Hills, CA: Sage.

Elliott, D. S., Huizinga, D., & Menard, S. (1989). *Multiple problem youth: Delinquency, substance use, and mental health problems.* New York: Springer-Verlag.

Epstein, N. B., Baldwin, L. M., & Bishop, D. S. (1983). The McMaster Family Assessment Device. *Journal of Marital and Family Therapy, 9,* 171–180.

Everington, C., & Dunn, C. (1995). A second validation study of the Competence Assessment for Standing Trial for Defendants with Mental Retardation (CAST-MR). *Criminal Justice and Behavior, 22,* 44–59.

Farnworth, M., Frazier, C. E., & Neuberger, A. R. (1988). Orientations to juvenile justice: Exploratory notes from a statewide survey of juvenile justice decisions makers. *Journal of Criminal Justice, 16,* 477–491.

Feldman, S. S., & Weinberger, D. A. (1994). Self-restraint as a mediator of family influences on boys' delinquent behavior: A longitudinal study. *Child Development, 65,* 195–211.

Floud, J., & Young, W. (1981). *Dangerousness and criminal justice.* London: Heinemann Educational Books.

Forth, A. E., & Brown, S. E. (1993). *The Antisocial Behaviours Scale.* Unpublished manuscript. Ottawa, Ontario: Carleton University.

Forth, A. E., Hart, S. D., & Hare, R. D. (1990). Assessment of psychopathology in male young offenders. *Psychological Assessment, 2,* 342–344.

Frazier, C. E., & Bishop, D. M. (1985). The pretrial detention of juveniles and its impact on case dispositions. *Journal of Criminal Law and Criminology, 76,* 1132–1152.

Freedman, B. J., Rosenthal, L., Donahoe, C. P., Schlundt, D. G., & McFall, R. M. (1978). A social–behavioral analysis of skill deficits in delinquent and nondelinquent adolescent boys. *Journal of Consulting and Clinical Psychology, 46,* 1448–1462.

Frick, P. J., O'Brien, B. S., Wooton, J. M., & McBurnett, K. (1994). Psychopathy and conduct problems in children. *Journal of Abnormal Psychology, 103,* 700–707.

Friedman, A. S., & Utada, A. (1989). A method for diagnosing and planning the treatment of adolescent drug abusers (The Adolescent Drug Abuse Diagnosis [ADAD] Interview). *Journal of Drug Education, 19,* 285–312.

Garb, H. N. (1989). Clinical judgment, clinical training, and professional experience. *Psychological Bulletin, 105,* 387–396.

Gardner, H. (1983). *Frames of mind: The theory of multiple intelligences.* New York: Basic Books.

Gardner, H., Krechevsky, M., Sternberg, R. J., & Okagaki, L. (1994). *Intelligence in context: Integrating cognitive theory and classroom practice.* Cambridge, MA: MIT Press.

Garner, D. M. (1996). The Eating Disorder Inventory–2. In L. I. Sederer & B. Dickey (Eds.), *Outcomes assessment in clinical practice* (pp. 92–96). Baltimore, MD: Williams & Wilkins.

Gendreau, P., & Andrews, D. A. (1994). *The Correctional Program Assessment Inventory.* St. John, New Brunswick: Department of Psychology, University of New Brunswick.

Gendreau, P., Grant, B. A., Leipciger, M., & Collins, C. (1979). Norms and recidivism rates for the MMPI and selected experimental scales on a Canadian delinquent sample. *Canadian Journal of Behavioural Science, 11,* 21–31.

Giller, H., & Tutt, N. (1987). Police cautioning of juveniles: The continuing practice of diversity. *Criminal Law Review,* 367–374.

Glaser, D. (1987). Classification for risk. In D. M. Gottfredson & M. Tonry (Eds.), *Prediction and classification: Criminal justice decision making* (pp. 249–292). Chicago: University of Chicago Press.

Gottfredson, M. R., & Gottfredson, D. M. (1988). *Decision making in criminal justice: Toward a rational exercise of discretion.* New York: Plenum Press.

Grisso, T. (1986). *Evaluating competencies: Forensic assessments and instruments.* New York: Plenum.

Grisso, T. (1987). The economic and scientific future of forensic assessment. *American Psychologist, 42,* 831–839.

Grisso, T., & Conlin, M. (1984). Procedural issues in the juvenile justice system. In N. Reppucci, L. Weithorn, E. Mulvey, & J. Monohan (Eds.), *Children, mental health, and the law* (pp. 171–193). Beverly Hills, CA: Sage.

Grisso, T., Tomkins, A., & Casey, P. (1988). Psychosocial concepts in juvenile law. *Law and Human Behavior, 12,* 403–437.

Guerra, N. G., Huesmann, L. R., & Hanish, L. (1994). The role of normative beliefs in children's social behavior. In N. Eisenberg (Ed.), *Social development* (pp. 140–158). Thousand Oaks, CA: Sage.

Gutterman, E. M., O'Brien, J. D., & Young, J. G. (1987). Structured diagnostic interviews for children and adolescents: Current status and future directions. *Journal of the American Academy of Child and Adolescent Psychiatry, 26,* 621–630.

Hallahan, D. P., & Kauffman, J. M. (1991). *Exceptional children: Introduction to special education* (5th ed.). Englewood Cliffs, NJ: Prentice-Hall.

Halleck, S. L., Hoge, S. K., Miller, R. D., Sadoff, R. L., & Halleck, N. H. (1992). The use of psychiatric diagnoses in the legal process: Task force report of the American Psychiatric Association. *Bulletin of the American Academy of Psychiatry and Law, 20,* 481–499.

Hammond, W. R., & Yung, B. (1993). Psychology's role in the public health response to assaultive violence among young African-American men. *American Psychologist, 48,* 142–154.

Hare, R. D. (1991). *The Psychopathy Checklist-Revised.* Toronto, Ontario: MHS Publishing.

Hare, R. D., Harpur, T. J., Hakstian, A. R., Forth, A. E., Hart, S. D., & Newman, J. P. (1990). The revised Psychopathy Checklist: Reliability and factor structure. *Psychological Assessment, 2,* 338–341.

Harris, M. M. (1989). Reconsidering the employment interview: A review of recent literature and suggestions for future research. *Personnel Psychology, 42,* 691–726.

Harris, P. M. (1988). Juvenile sentence reform and its evaluation. *Evaluation Review, 12,* 655–666.

Harris, P. W. (1988). The Interpersonal Maturity Level Classification System. *Criminal Justice and Behavior, 15,* 58–77.

Hart, S. D., Webster, C. D., & Menzies, R. J. (1993). A note on portraying the accuracy of violence predictions. *Law and Human Behavior, 17,* 695–700.

Hawkins, J. D., & Catalano, R. F. (1992). *Communities that care.* San Francisco, CA: Jossey-Bass.

Hawkins, J. D., Catalano, R. F., & Brewer, D. D. (1995). Preventing serious, violent, and chronic juvenile offending: Effective strategies from conception to age 6. In J. C. Howell, B. Krisberg, J. D. Hawkins, & J. J. Wilson (Eds.), *A sourcebook: Serious, violent, and chronic juvenile offenders* (pp. 47–60). Thousand Oaks, CA: Sage.

Hawkins, J. D., Catalano, R. F., & Miller, J. Y. (1992). Risk and protective factors for alcohol and other drug problems in adolescence and early adulthood: Implications for substance abuse prevention. *Psychological Bulletin, 112,* 64–105.

Henggeler, S. W. (1989). *Delinquency in adolescence.* Newbury Park, CA: Sage.

Henggeler, S. W. (1991). Multidimensional models of delinquent behavior and their implications for treatment. In R. Cohen & A. W. Siegel (Eds.), *Context and development* (pp. 211–231). Hillsdale, NJ: Erlbaum.

Henggeler, S. W., Melton, G. B., & Smith, L. A. (1992). Family preservation using multisystemic therapy: An effective alternative to incarcerating serious juvenile offenders. *Journal of Consulting and Clinical Psychology, 60,* 953–961.

Henggeler, S. W., Melton, G. B., Smith, L. A., Schoenwald, S. K., & Hanley, J. H. (1993). Family preservation using multisystematic treatment: Long term follow-up to a clinical trial with serious juvenile offenders. *Journal of Child and Family Studies, 2,* 283–293.

Herjanic, B., Herjanic, M., Brown, F., and Wheatt, T. (1975). Are children reliable reporters? *Journal of Abnormal Child Psychology, 3,* 41–48.

Hersen, M., & Ammerman, R. T. (1995). *Advanced abnormal child psychology.* Hillsdale, NJ: Erlbaum.

Hirschi, T., & Hindelang, M. V. (1977). Intelligence and delinquency: A revisionist review. *American Sociological Review, 42,* 571–587.

Hodges, K. (1985). *Manual for the Child Assessment Schedule.* Ypsilanti, MI: Department of Psychology, Eastern Michigan University.

Hodges, K. (1993). Structured interviews for assessing children. *Journal of Child Psychology and Psychiatry, 34,* 49–68.

Hodges, K., Cools, J., & McKnew, D. (1989). Test-retest reliability of a clinical research interview for children: The Child Assessment Schedule. *Psychological Assessment, 1,* 317–322.

Hoge, R. D. (1983). Psychometric properties of teacher-judgment measures of pupil aptitudes, classroom behaviors, and achievement levels. *Journal of Special Education, 17,* 401–429.

Hoge, R. D., & Andrews, D. A. (1986). A model for conceptualizing interventions in social service agencies. *Canadian Psychology, 27,* 332–341.

Hoge, R. D., & Andrews, D. A. (1992). Assessing conduct problems in the classroom. *Clinical Psychology Review, 12,* 1–20.

Hoge, R. D., & Andrews, D. A. (1994). *The Youth Level of Service/Case Management Inventory and manual.* Ottawa, Ontario: Department of Psychology, Carleton University.

Hoge, R. D., & Andrews, D. A. (1996, August). *Assessing risk and need factors in the youthful offender.* Presentation at the Annual Conference of the American Psychological Association, Toronto, Ontario.

Hoge, R. D., Andrews, D. A., & Leschied, A. W. (1994). Tests of three hypotheses regarding the predictors of delinquency. *Journal of Abnormal Child Psychology, 22,* 547–559.

Hoge, R. D., Andrews, D. A., & Leschied, A. W. (1995). Investigation of variables asssociated with probation and custody dispositions in a sample of juveniles. *Journal of Clinical Child Psychology, 24,* 279–286.

Hoge, R. D., Andrews, D. A., & Leschied, A. W. (1996). An investigation of risk and protective factors in a sample of youthful offenders. *Journal of Child Psychology and Psychiatry, 37,* 419–424.

Hoge, R. D., & Coladarci, T. (1989). Teacher-based judgments of academic achievement: A review of literature. *Review of Educational Research, 59,* 297–313.

Hoge, R. D., & Renzulli, J. S. (1993). Exploring the link between giftedness and self-concept. *Review of Educational Research, 63,* 449–465.

Holden, G. W., & Edwards, L. A. (1989). Parental attitudes toward child rearing: Instruments, issues, and implications. *Psychological Bulletin, 106,* 29–58.

Hunt, D. E. (1971). *Matching models in education.* Toronto: Ontario Institute for Studies in Education.

Hunt, D. E., Butler, L. F., Noy, J. E., & Rosser, M. E. (1971). *Assessing conceptual level by the paragraph completion method.* Toronto: Ontario Institute for Studies in Education.

Jackson, D. N. (1994). *The Jackson Vocational Interest Survey Manual.* Port Huron, MI: Sigma Assessment Systems, Inc.

Jackson, D. N. (1995). *The Basic Personality Inventory Manual.* Port Huron, MI: Sigma Assessment Systems, Inc.

Jackson, D. N., Helmes, E., Hoffmann, H., Holden, R. R., Jaffe, P. G., Reddon, J. R., & Smiley, W. C. (1989). *The Basic Personality Inventory Manual.* Port Huron, MI: Sigma Assessment Systems.

Jacob, T., & Tennenbaum, D. L. (1988). *Family assessment: Rationale, methods, and future directions.* New York: Plenum.

Jaffe, P. G., Leschied, A. W., Sas, L., & Austin, G. W. (1985). A model for the provision of clinical assessments and service brokerage for young offenders: The London Family Court Clinic. *Canadian Psychology, 26,* 54–61.

Jesness, C. F., & Wedge, R. F. (1984). Validity of a revised Jesness Inventory I-Level classification with delinquents. *Journal of Consulting and Clinical Psychology, 52,* 997–1010.

Jesness, C. F., & Wedge, R. F. (1985). *Jesness Inventory classification system: Supplementary manual.* Palo Alto, CA: Consulting Psychologists Press.

Jessor, R., Donovan, J. E., & Costa, F. M. (1991). *Beyond adolescence: Problem behavior and young adult development.* Cambridge: Cambridge University Press.

Jessor, R., & Jessor, S. L. (1977). *Problem behavior and psychosocial development: A longitudinal study of youth.* New York: Academic Press.

Kaufman, A. S. (1979). *Intelligent testing with the WISC-R.* New York: Wiley.

Kaufman, A. S., & Kaufman, N. L. (1985). *Kaufman Test of Educational Achievement.* Circle Pines, MN: American Guidance Service.

Kazdin, A. E. (1987). *Conduct disorders in childhood and adolescence.* Newbury Park, CA: Sage.

Kazdin, A. E. (1989). Developmental psychopathology: Current research, issues, and directions. *American Psychologist, 44,* 180–187.

Kazdin, A. E. (1993). Adolescent mental health: Prevention and treatment programs. *American Psychologist, 48,* 127–141.

Kazdin, A. E., & Esveldt-Dawson, K. (1986). The Interview for Antisocial Behavior: Psychometric characteristics and concurrent validity with child psychiatric inpatients. *Journal of Psychopathology and Behavioral Assessment, 8,* 289–303.

Keyser, D. J., & Sweetland, R. C. (1992). *Test critiques.* Kansas City, MO: Test Corporation of America.

Knight, R. A., & Prentky, R. (1993). Exploring characteristics for classifying juvenile sex offenders. In H. E. Barbaree, W. L. Marshall, & S. M. Hudson (Eds.), *The juvenile sex offender* (pp. 45–83). New York: Guilford.

Kolb, B., & Whishaw, I. Q. (1985). *Fundamentals of human neuropsychology* (2nd ed.). New York: Freeman.

Kolko, D. J., & Kazdin, A. E. (1989). Assessment of dimensions of childhood firesetting among patients and nonpatients: The Firesetting Risk Interview. *Journal of Abnormal Child Psychology, 17,* 157–176.

Kravitz, D. A., Cutler, B. L., & Brock, P. (1993). Reliability and validity of the original and revised Legal Attitudes Questionnaire. *Law and Human Behavior, 17,* 661–667.

L'Abate, L., & Bagarozzi, D. A. (1993). *Sourcebook of marriage and family evaluation.* New York: Brunner/Mazel.

Lachar, D., & Kline, R. B. (1994). Personality Inventory for Children and Personality Inventory for Youth. In M. E. Maruish (Ed.), *The use of psychological testing for treatment planning and outcome assessment* (pp. 479–516). Hillsdale, NJ: Erlbaum.

Lanyon, R. (1984). Personality assessment. *Annual Review of Psychology, 35,* 689–701.

Last, C. G. (1987). Developmental considerations. In C. G. Last & M. Hersen (Eds.), *Issues in diagnostic research* (pp. 201–216). New York: Plenum.

Le Blanc, B., & Beaumont, H. (1992). The effectiveness of juvenile justice in Quebec: A natural experiment in implementing formal diversion and a justice model. In R. R. Corrado, N. Bala, R. Linden, & M. Le Blanc (Eds.), *Juvenile justice in Canada: A theoretical and analytical assessment* (pp. 283–312). Toronto: Butterworths.

Le Blanc, B., Ouimet, M., & Tremblay, R. E. (1988). An integrative control theory of delinquent behavior: A validation of 1976–1985. *Psychiatry, 51,* 164–176.

Leschied, A. W., Austin, G. W., & Jaffe, P. G. (1988). Impact of the Young Offenders Act on recidivism rates of special needs youth: Clinical and policy implications. *Canadian Journal of Behavioural Science, 20,* 322–331.

Leschied, A. W., Jaffe, P. G., Andrews, D. A., & Gendreau, P. (1992). Treatment issues and young offenders: An empirically derived vision of juvenile justice policy. In R. R. Corrado, N. Bala, R.

Linden, & M. Le Blanc (Eds.), *Juvenile justice in Canada: A theoretical and analytical assessment* (pp. 347–366). Toronto: Butterworths.

Lezak, M. D. (1995). *Neuropsychological assessment*. New York: Oxford University Press.

Lipsey, M. W., & Wilson, D. B. (1993). The efficacy of psychological, educational, and behavioral treatments: Confirmation from meta-analysis. *American Psychologist, 48,* 1181–1209.

Loeber, R., & Dishion, T. J. (1983). Early predictors of male delinquency: A review. *Psychological Bulletin, 94,* 68–99.

Loeber, R., Dishion, T. J., & Patterson, G. R. (1984). Multiple gating: A multistage assessment procedure for identifying youths at risk for delinquency. *Journal of Research in Crime and Delinquency, 21,* 7–32.

Loeber, R., Keenan, K., Lahey, B. B., Green, S. M., & Thomas, C. (1993). Evidence for developmentally based diagnoses of oppositional defiant disorder and conduct disorder. *Journal of Abnormal Child Psychology, 21,* 377–410.

Loeber, R., & Stouthamer-Loeber, M. (1986). Family factors as correlates and predictors of juvenile conduct problems and delinquency. In M. Tonry & N. Morris (Eds.), *Crime and justice: An annual review of research* (Vol. 7, pp. 29–150). Chicago: University of Chicago Press.

Loeber, R., & Stouthamer-Loeber, M. (1987). Prediction. In H. C. Quay (Ed.), *Handbook of juvenile delinquency* (pp. 325–382). New York: Wiley.

Loeber, R., & Stouthamer-Loeber, M. (1996). The development of offending. *Criminal Justice and Behavior, 23,* 12–24.

Luthar, S. S. (1993). Annotation: Methodological and conceptual issues in research on childhood resilience. *Journal of Child Psychology and Psychiatry, 14,* 441–453.

Mak, A. S. (1993). A self-report delinquency scale for Australian adolescents. *Australian Journal of Psychology, 45,* 75–79.

Markwart, A. (1992). Custodial sanctions under the young offenders Act. In R. R. Corrado, N. Bala, R. Linden, & M. Le Blanc (Eds.), *Juvenile justice in Canada: A theoretical and analytical assessment* (pp. 229–281). Toronto: Butterworths.

Marsh, H. W., & O'Neill, R. (1984). Self Description Questionnaire III: The construct validity of multidimensional self-concept ratings by late adolescents. *Journal of Educational Measurement, 21,* 153–174.

Mash, E. J., & Terdal, L. G. (1988). *Behavioral assessment of childhood disorders*. New York: Guilford.

Matarazzo, J. D. (1986). Computerized clinical psychological test interpretations: Unvalidated plus all mean and no sigma. *American Psychologist, 41,* 14–24.

Matarazzo, J. D. (1990). Psychological assessment versus psychological testing: Validation from Binet to the school, clinic, and courtroom. *American Psychologist, 45,* 999–1017.

McConaughy, S. H., & Achenbach, T. M. (1990). *Guide for the Semistructured Clinical Interview for Children Aged 6–11*. Burlington, VT: University of Vermont, Department of Psychiatry.

McDermott, J. (1983). The serious juvenile offender: Problems in definition and targeting. In J. R. Klugel (Ed.), *Evaluating juvenile justice* (pp. 67–90). Beverly Hills, CA: Sage.

McDermott, P. A., Marston, N. C., & Stott, D. H. (1993). *Adjustment scales for children and adolescents*. Philadelphia, PA: Edumetric and Clinical Science.

McReynolds, P. (1989). Diagnosis and clinical assessment: Current status and major issues. *Annual Review of Psychology, 40,* 83–108.

Megargee, E. I. (1977). A new classification system for criminal offenders. *Criminal Justice and Behavior, 4,* 107–114.

Megargee, E. I. (1984). A new classification system for criminal offenders: VI: Differences among the types on the adjective checklist. *Criminal Justice and Behavior, 11,* 349–376.

Megargee, E. I., & Bohn, M. (1979). *Classifying criminal offenders: A new system based on the MMPI.* Beverly Hills, CA: Sage.

Melton, G. B., Petrila, J., Poythress, N. G., & Slobogin, C. (1987). *Psychological evaluations for the court: A handbook for mental health professionals and lawyers.* New York: Guilford.

Messick, S. (1989a). Validity. In R. L. Linn (Ed.), *Educational measurement* (3rd ed., pp. 13–103). Washington, DC: American Council on Education and National Council on Measurement in Education.

Messick, S. (1989b). Meaning and values in test validation: The science and ethics of assessment. *Educational Researcher, 18,* 5–11.

Messick, S. (1995). Validity of psychological assessment: Validation of inferences from persons' responses and performances as scientific inquiry into score meaning. *American Psychologist, 50,* 741–749.

Meyer, R. G., & Deitsch, S. E. (1996). *The clinician's handbook: Integrated diagnostics, assessment, and in adult and adolescent psychopathology* (4th ed.). New York: Allyn & Bacon.

Millon, T., Green, C. J., & Meagher, R. B. (1982). *Millon Adolescent Personality Inventory manual.* Minneapolis, MN: National Computer Systems.

Moos, R. H. (1975). *Evaluating correctional and community settings.* New York: Wiley.

Moos, R. H. (1986a). *Correctional Institutions Environment Scale manual* (2nd ed.). Palo Alto, CA: Consulting Psychologists Press.

Moos, R. H. (1986b). *Community-Oriented Programs Environment Scale manual.* Palo Alto, CA: Consulting Psychologists Press.

Moos, R. H., & Moos, B. (1986). *The Family Environment Scale manual* (2nd ed.). Palo Alto, CA: Consulting Psychologists Press.

Morris, A., & Giller, H. (1987). *Understanding juvenile justice.* London: Croom Helm.

Mrazek, D. A., Mrazek, P., & Klinnert, M. (1995). Clinical assessment of parenting. *Journal of the American Academy of Child and Adolescent Psychiatry, 34,* 272–282.

Mulvey, E. P. (1984). Judging amenability to treatment in juvenile offenders: Theory and practice. In N. Reppucci, L. Weithorn, E. Mulvey, & J. Monohan (Eds.), *Children, mental health, and the law* (pp. 195–210). Beverly Hills, CA: Sage.

Mulvey, E. P., Arthur, M. W., & Reppucci, N. D. (1993). The prevention and treatment of juvenile delinquency: A review of research. *Clinical Psychology Review, 13,* 133–167.

Murphy, K. R., & Davidshofer, C. O. (1988). *Psychological testing: Principles and applications.* Englewood Cliffs, NJ: Prentice-Hall.

Niarhos, F. J., & Routh, D. K. (1992). The role of clinical assessment in the juvenile court: Predictors of juvenile dispositions and recidivism. *Journal of Clinical Child Psychology, 21,* 151–159.

Olson, D. H., Partner, J., & Lavoie, Y. (1985). *FACES III.* St. Paul, MN: University of Minnesota Publications.

Overall, J. E., & Pfefferbaum, B. (1982). The Brief Psychiatric Rating Scale for Children. *Psychopharmacology Bulletin, 18,* 10–16.

Palmer, T. (1984). Treatment and the role of classification: A review of basics. *Crime and Delinquency, 30,* 245–267.

Palmer, T. (1992). *The re-emergence of correctional interventions.* Newbury Park, CA: Sage.

Palmer, T. (1994). *A profile of correctional effectiveness and new directions for research.* Albany, NY: State University of New York Press.

Patterson, G. R., DeBaryshe, B. D., & Ramsey, E. (1989). A developmental persepective on antisocial behavior. *American Psychologist, 44,* 329–335.

Patterson, G. R., Reid, J. B., & Dishion, T. J. (1992). *Antisocial boys.* Eugene, OR: Castalia.

Pratt, J. (1989). Corporatism: The third model of juvenile justice. *British Journal of Criminology, 29,* 236–253.

Quay, H. C. (1964). Personality dimensions in delinquent males as inferred from the factor analysis of behavior ratings. *Journal of Research in Crime and Delinquency, 1,* 33–37.

Quay, H. C. (1966). Personality patterns in preadolescent delinquent boys. *Educational and Psychological Measurement, 16,* 99–110.

Quay, H. C. (1987). Patterns of delinquent behavior. In H. C. Quay (Ed.), *Handbook of juvenile delinquency* (pp. 118–138). New York: Wiley.

Quay, H. C., & Peterson, D. R. (1987). *Manual for the Revised Behavior Problem Checklist.* Miami, FL: University of Miami.

Quay, H. C., Routh, D. K., & Shapiro, S. K. (1987). Psychopathology of childhood: From description to evaluation. *Annual Review of Psychology, 38,* 491–532.

Raven, J. C., Court, J. H., & Raven, J. (1986). *Raven's progressive matrices and vocabularly scales.* London: Lewis.

Reid, S. A., & Reitsma-Street, M. (1984). Assumptions and implications of new Canadian legislation for young offenders. *Canadian Criminology Forum, 17,* 334–352.

Reitan, R. M., & Wolfson, D. (1985). *The Halstead-Reitan Neuropsychological Test Battery.* Tuscon, AZ: Neuropsychology Press.

Reitsma-Street, M. (1991). A review of female delinquency. In A. W. Leschied, P. G. Jaffe, & W. Willis (Eds.), *The Young Offenders Act: A revolution in Canadian juvenile justice* (pp. 248–287). Toronto: University of Toronto Press.

Reitsma-Street, M., & Leschied, A. W. (1988). The Conceptual-Level Matching Model in corrections. *Criminal Justice and Behavior, 15,* 92–108.

Reynolds, C. R., & Kamphaus, R. W. (1992). *Manual: Behavior Assessment System for Children.* Circle Pines, MN: American Guidance Service.

Rigby, K. (1982). A concise scale for the assessment of attitudes toward institutional authority. *Australian Journal of Psychology, 34,* 195–204.

Robin, A. L., Koepke, T., & Moye, A. (1990). Multidimensional assessment of parent-adolescent relations. *Psychological Assessment, 2,* 451–459.

Roehling, P. V., & Robin, A. (1986). Development and validation of the Family Beliefs Inventory: A measure of unrealistic beliefs among parents and adolescents. *Journal of Consulting and Clinical Psychology, 54,* 693–697.

Roesch, R., & Golding, S. L. (1987). Defining and assessing competency to stand trial. In I. B. Weiner & A. K. Hess (Eds.), *Handbook of forensic psychology* (pp. 378–394). New York: Wiley.

Roesch, R., Ogloff, J. R. P., & Golding, S. L. (1993). Competency to stand trial: Legal and clinical issues. *Applied and Preventive Psychology, 2,* 43–51.

Roesch, R., Webster, C. D., & Eaves, D. (1984). *The Fitness Interview Test: A method for examining fitness to stand trial.* Toronto: Centre of Criminology, University of Toronto.

Rogers, R., & Mitchell, C. N. (1991). *Mental health experts and the criminal courts.* Toronto: Carswell Publications.

Rotatori, A. F. (1994). Multidimensional Self Concept Scale. *Measurement and Evaluation in Counseling and Development, 26,* 265–268.

Rutter, M. (1987). Psychosocial resilience and protective mechanisms. *American Journal of Orthopsychiatry, 57,* 316–331.

Rutter, M. (1990). Psychosocial resilience and protective mechanisms. In J. Rolf, A. S. Masten, D. Cicchetti, K. H. Nuechterlien, & S. Weintraub (Eds.), *Risk and protective factors in the development of psychopathology* (pp. 181–214). New York: Cambridge University Press.

Sattler, J. M. (1992). *Assessment of children* (3rd ed., rev.). San Diego, CA: Author.

Sbordone, R. J. (1991). *Neuropsychology for the attorney.* Orlando, FL: Paul M. Deutsch Press.

Schaefer, E. (1965). Children's reports of parental behavior: An inventory. *Child Development, 36,* 413–424.

Schissel, B. (1993). *Social dimensions of Canadian youth justice.* Toronto: Oxford University Press.

Schluderman, E., & Schluderman, S. (1970). Replicability of factors in Children's Report of Parental Behavior Inventory (CRPBI). *Journal of Psychology, 76,* 239–249.

Schluderman, S., & Schluderman, E. (1983). Sociocultural change and adolescents' perceptions of parent behavior. *Developmental Psychology, 19*, 674–685.

Sellin, T., & Wolfgang, M. E. (1964). *The measurement of delinquency.* New York: Wiley.

Shaffer, D., Schwab-Stone, M., Fisher, P., Cohen, P., Piacentini, J., Davies, M., Conners, C. K., & Regier, D. (1993). The Diagnostic Interview Schedule for Children Revised Versions (DISC-R): Preparation, field testing, inter-rater reliability and acceptability. *Journal of the American Academy of Child and Adolescent Psychiatry, 32*, 643–650.

Shaw, M. W., & Wright, M. (1967). *Scales for the measurement of attitudes.* New York: McGraw-Hill.

Shields, I. W., & Simourd, D. J. (1991). Predicting predatory behavior in a population of young offenders. *Criminal Justice and Behavior, 18*, 180–194.

Shields, I. W., & Whitehall, G. C. (1991). *The Pride in Delinquency Scale.* Ottawa, Ontario: Department of Psychology, Carleton University.

Shields, I. W., & Whitehall, G. C. (1994). Neutralization and delinquency among teenagers. *Criminal Justice and Behavior, 21*, 223–235.

Siassi, I. (1984). Psychiatric interview and mental status examination. In G. Goldstein & H. Hersen (Eds.), *Handbook of psychological assessment* (pp. 259–275). New York: Pergamon.

Silvaroli, N. J. (1986). *Classroom Reading Inventory* (5th ed.). Dubuque, IA: Wm. C. Brown.

Simourd, D. J. (in press). The Criminal Sentiments Scale-Modified and Pride in Delinquency Scale. *Criminal Justice and Behavior.*

Simourd, D. J., Hoge, R. D., Andrews, D. A., & Leschied, A. W. (1994). An empirically-based typology of male young offenders. *Canadian Journal of Criminology, 36*, 447–461.

Skinner, H. A., & Sheu, W. J. (1982). Reliability of alcohol use indices: The Lifetime Drinking History and the MAST. *Studies on Alcohol, 43*, 1157–1170.

Snow, R. E. (1991). Aptitude-treatment interaction as a framework for research on individual differences in psychotherapy. *Journal of Consulting and Clinical Psychology, 59*, 205–216.

Sparrow, S. S., Balla, D. A., & Cicchetti, D. V. (1984). *Vineland Adaptive Behavior Scales.* Circle Pines, MN: American Guidance Service.

Stanford, M. S., Ebner, D., Patton, J. H., & Williams, J. (1994). Multi-impulsivity within an adolescent psychiatric population. *Personality and Individual Differences, 16*, 395–402.

Sternberg, R. (1985). *Beyond IQ: A triarchic theory of human intelligence.* Cambridge: Cambridge University Press.

Sternberg, R. (1988). *The triarchic mind: A new theory of human intelligence.* New York: Cambridge University Press.

Strayhorn, J. M., & Weidman, C. S. (1988). A parent practices scale and its relation to parent and child mental health. *Journal of the American Academy of Child and Adolescent Psychiatry, 27*, 613–618.

Tarter, R. E. (1990). Evaluation and treatment of adolescent substance abuse: A decision tree method. *American Journal of Drug and Alcohol Abuse, 16*, 1–46.

Tate, D. C., Reppucci, N. D., & Mulvey, E. P. (1995). Violent juvenile delinquents: Treatment effectiveness and implications for future action. *American Psychologist, 50*, 777–781.

Thomas, C. W., & Fitch, S. M. (1981). The exercise of discretion in the juvenile justice system. *Juvenile and Family Court Journal, 32*, 31–50.

Thornberry, T. P., Huizinga, D., & Loeber, R. (1995). The prevention of serious delinquency and violence: Implications from the program of research on the causes and correlates of delinquency. In J. C. Howell, B. Krisberg, J. D. Hawkins, & J. J. Wilson (Eds.), *A sourcebook: Serious, violent, and chronic juvenile offenders* (pp. 213–237). Thousand Oaks, CA: Sage.

Touliatos, J., Perlmutter, B. F., & Straus, M. A. (1990). *Handbook of family measurement techniques.* Newbury Park, CA: Sage.

Tremblay, R. E. (1992). The predictors of delinquent behavior from childhood behavior: Personality theory revisited. In J. McCord (Ed.), *Facts, frameworks, and forecasts: Advances in criminological theory* (pp. 193–230). New Brunswick, NJ: Transaction Publishers.

Trevethan, S. D., & Walker, L. J. (1989). Hypothetical vs real-life moral reasoning among psychopathic and delinquent youth. *Development and Psychopathology, 1,* 91–103.

Valcuikas, J. A. (1995). *Forensic neuropsychology: Conceptual foundations and clinical practice.* New York: Haworth Press.

Van Voorhis, P. (1994). *Psychological classification of the adult male prison inmate.* Albany, NY: State University of New York Press.

Vaneziano, C., & Vaneziano, L. (1986). Classification of adolescent offenders with the MMPI: An extension and cross-validation of the Megargee typology. *International Journal of Offender Therapy and Comparative Criminology, 30,* 4–23.

Vold, G. V., & Bernard, T. J. (1986). *Theoretical criminology* (3rd ed.). Oxford: Oxford University Press.

Waldman, I. D., Lilienfield, S. O., & Lahey, B. B. (1995). Toward construct validity in the childhood disruptive behavior disorders: Classification and diagnosis in DSM-IV and beyond. *Advances in Clinical Child Psychology, 17,* 323–363.

Warren, M. Q. (1966). *Interpersonal maturity level classification: Juvenile diagnosis and treatment of low, middle, and high maturity delinquents.* Sacramento, CA: California Youth Authority.

Warren, M. Q. (1976). Intervention with juvenile delinquents. In M. Rosenheim (Ed.), *Pursuing justice for the child.* Chicago: University of Chicago Press.

Warren, M. Q. (1983). Applications of interpersonal-maturity theory to offender populations. In W. S. Laufer & J. M. Day (Eds.), *Personality theory, moral development, and criminal behavior* (pp. 23–50). Lexington, MA: Lexington Books.

Webster, C. D., Rogers, J. M., Cochrane, J. J., & Stylianos, S. (1991). Assessment and treatment of mentally disordered young offenders. In A. W. Leschied, P. G. Jaffe, & W. Willis (Eds.), *The Young Offenders Act: A revolution in Canadian juvenile justice* (pp. 197–229). Toronto, Ont.: University of Toronto Press.

Wechsler, D. (1981). *Wechsler Adult Intelligence Scale-Revised.* San Antonio, TX: The Psychological Corporation.

Wechsler, D. (1991). *Wechsler Intelligence Scale for Children-III.* San Antonio, TX: The Psychological Corporation.

Weisstub, D. (1984). *Law and mental health: International perspectives.* New York: Pergamon Press.

Werry, J. S. (1992). Child psychiatric disorders: Are they classifiable? *British Journal of Psychiatry, 161,* 472–480.

Wiebush, R. G., Baird, C., Krisberg, B., & Onek, D. (1995). Risk assessment and classification for serious, violent, and chronic juvenile offenders. In J. C. Howell, B. F. Krisberg, J. D. Hawkins, & J. J. Wilson (Eds.), *A sourcebook: Serious, violent, and chronic juvenile offenders* (pp. 171–212). Thousand Oaks, CA: Sage.

Woodward, M. J., Goncalves, A. A., & Millon, T. (1994). Millon Personality Inventory and Millon Adolescent Clinical Inventory. In M. E. Maruish (Ed.), *The use of psychological testing for treatment planning and outcome assessment* (pp. 453–478). Hillsdale, NJ: Erlbaum.

Woolard, J. L., Gross, S. L., Mulvey, E. P., & Reppucci, N. D. (1992). Legal issues affecting mentally disordered youth in the juvenile justice system. In J. J. Cocozza (Ed.), *Responding to the mental health needs of youth in the juvenile justice system* (pp. 91–106). Seattle, WA: National Coalition for the Mentally Ill in the Criminal Justice System.

Wormith, J. S. (1995). The Youth Management Assessment: Assessment of young offenders at risk of serious reoffending. *Forum, 7,* 23–27.

Wright, K. N. (1985). Developing the Prison Environment Inventory. *Journal of Research in Crime and Delinquency, 22,* 257–277.

Yoshikawa, H. (1994). Prevention as cumulative protection: Effects of early family support and education on chronic delinquency and its risks. *Psychological Bulletin, 115,* 28–54.

Zager, L. D. (1988). The MMPI-based criminal classification sysem: A review, current status, and future directions. *Criminal Justice and Behavior, 15,* 39–57.

Author Index

Abikoff, H., 64, 117
Achenbach, T. M., 60, 63, 64.
   72, 73, 104, 117, 124
Ageton, S. S., 8, 69, 119, 120
Akers, R. L., 8, 117
American Psychiatric Association, 80, 81, 117
American Psychological Association, 31, 32, 42, 101,
   117
Ammerman, R. T., 106, 122
Anastasi, A., 34, 117
Andrews, D. A., 8, 9, 11, 12,
   13, 23, 24, 26–27, 37,
   52, 60, 65, 66, 69, 74,
   75, 76, 79, 87, 90, 92,
   94, 95, 101, 105, 106,
   107, 117, 120, 122,
   123–124, 127
Archer, R. P., 82, 93, 117,
   118
Arthur, M. W., 106, 125
Ashford, J. B., 87, 88, 94, 95,
   117, 118
August, G. J., 105, 118
Austin, G. W., 56, 104, 109,
   122, 123

Bagarozzi, D. A., 70, 75–76,
   123
Baird, S. C., 22, 79, 85, 87,
   89, 100, 118, 128
Bala, N., 17, 118
Baldwin, L. M., 71, 120
Balla, D. A., 61, 62, 127
Beaulieu, L. A., 24, 26
Beaumont, H., 4, 123
Bennett, B. E., 32, 104, 119
Bennett, L. A., 104, 118
Ben-Porath, Y. S., 82, 118
Bernard, T. J., 128

Beutler, L. E., 76, 118
Billings, A., 71, 118
Binder, A., 24, 26, 79, 118
Bishop, D. M., 16, 120
Bishop, D. S., 71, 120
Blaske, D. M., 69, 75, 118
Bohn, M., 81, 124
Bond-Maupin, L., 66, 87, 88,
   95, 106, 118
Bonta, J., 8, 9, 11, 12, 23, 37,
   52, 65, 66, 69, 75, 79,
   87, 90, 92, 94, 95, 106,
   107, 117
Borduin, C. M., 69, 75, 118
Brewer, D. D., 8, 107, 121
Brock, P., 64, 123
Brodsky, S. L., 65, 118
Bronfenbrenner, U., 69, 118
Brown, F., 61, 62, 122
Bruce, D., 24, 79, 118
Bruininks, R. H., 62, 118
Butcher, J. N., 82, 118
Butler, J. W., 73, 118
Butler, L. F., 83, 122
Byrne, B. M., 58, 118

Campbell, D. T., 35, 118
Canadian Psychological Asso-
   ciation, 32, 118
Canter, R. J., 32, 119
Carrington, P. J., 24, 119
Carrow-Woolfolk, E., 47,
   119
Casey, P., 26, 121
Catalano, R. F., 8, 12, 65,
   106, 107, 121
Champion, D. J., 79, 85, 87,
   119
Chan, J. B. L., 16, 24, 119
Cicchetti, D. V., 61, 62, 127
Clarkin, J., 76, 118

Clear, T., 22, 119
Clements, C. B., 22, 79, 119
Cline, T., 25, 119
Cochrane, J. J., 21, 128
Cohen, P., 62, 63, 105, 127
Cohen, S., 119
Coladarci, T., 25, 72, 122
Collins, C., 64, 65, 120
Cone, L. T., 75, 118
Conlin, M., 17, 24, 121
Conners, C. K., 127
Conoley, J. C., 42, 103, 119
Cools, J., 63, 122
Copmas, B. E., 119
Corrado, R. R., 3, 4, 5, 6, 24,
   25, 119
Costa, F. M., 8, 123
Costello, E. J., 62, 63, 119
Court, J. H., 46, 126
Crealock, C. M., 52, 119
Crosby, R. D., 105, 118
Cutler, D. L., 64, 123

Dannefer, D., 24, 119
Davidshofer, C. O., 62, 125
Davies, M., 62, 63, 105, 127
Dawes, R. M., 25, 119
DeBaryshe, B. D., 99, 125
Deitsch, S. E., 55, 125
Dishion, T. J., 12, 37, 71,
   99–100, 105, 124, 125
Donahoe, C. P., 63–64, 120
Donovan, J. E., 8, 123
Doob, A. N., 16, 24, 26, 119
Dulcan, M. K., 62, 119
Dunn, C., 92, 120

Eaves, D., 92, 126
Ebner, D., 88, 127
Edelbrock, L. S., 62, 119
Edwards, L. A., 75–76, 122

Elliott, D. S., 8, 61, 69, 119, 120
Epstein, N. B., 120
Esveldt-Dawson, K., 63, 64, 123
Everington, C., 92, 120

Farnsworth, M., 25–26, 120
Faust, D., 25, 119
Feldman, S. S., 72, 99–100, 120
Fisher, P., 62, 63, 105, 127
Fiske, D. W., 35, 118
Fitch, S. M., 24, 127
Floud, J., 85, 120
Forshag, H., 104, 118
Forth, A. E., 61, 88, 90, 120, 121
Frazier, C. E., 16, 25–26, 120
Freedman, B. J., 63–64, 120
Frick, P. J., 90, 120
Friedman, A. S., 63–64, 120
Fucci, B. R., 75, 118

Garb, H. N., 25, 62, 120
Gardner, H., 46–47, 120
Garner, D. M., 61, 120
Gates, G., 73, 118
Geis, G., 24, 79, 118
Gendreau, P., 24, 64, 65, 74, 120, 123–124
Gerhardt, C. A., 119
Giller, H., 8, 16, 120, 125
Gittelman, R., 64, 117
Glaser, D., 22, 120
Golding, S. L., 108, 126
Goncalves, A. A., 56, 128
Gottfredson, D. M., 24, 40, 120
Gottfredson, M. R., 24, 40, 120
Graham, J. R., 82, 118
Grant, B. A., 64, 65, 120
Green, C. J., 56, 57, 125
Green, S. M., 107, 124
Grisso, T., 17, 24, 26, 32, 35, 39, 41, 53, 92, 99, 103, 108, 121
Gross, S. L., 21, 128
Guerra, N. G., 65, 121
Gutterman, E. M., 62, 63, 81, 121

Hakstian, A.R., 88, 121
Hallahan, D. P., 61–62, 121
Halleck, N. H., 41, 53, 121
Halleck, S. L., 35, 53, 121
Hammond, W. R., 109, 121
Hanish, L., 65, 121
Hanley, J. H., 75, 121
Hare, R. D., 30, 64, 88, 90, 95, 101, 120, 121
Harpur, T. J., 88, 121
Harris, M. M., 25, 121
Harris, P. W., 82–83, 121
Hart, S. D., 37, 38, 90, 120, 121
Hawkins, J. D., 8, 12, 65, 106, 107, 121
Helmes, E., 122
Henggeler, S. W., 8, 12, 69, 75, 99, 106, 118, 121
Herjanic, B., 62, 122
Herjanic, M., 62, 122
Hersen, M., 106, 122
Hill, B. K., 62, 118
Hindelang, M. V., 52, 122
Hinden, B. R., 119
Hirschi, T., 52, 122
Hodges, K., 62, 63, 122
Hoffmann, H., 122
Hoge, R. D., 8, 12, 13, 24, 25, 26–27, 35, 41, 53, 58, 60, 72, 76, 87, 90, 92, 95, 101, 105, 107, 117, 122, 127
Holden, G. W., 75–76, 122
Huartson, K., 92, 117
Huesmann, L., 65, 121
Huizinga, D., 8, 61, 69, 106, 119, 120, 127
Hunt, D.E ., 83, 122

Impara, J. C., 41, 103, 119

Jackson, D. N., 49, 56, 104, 107, 122
Jacob, T., 70, 122
Jaffe, P. G., 24, 56, 104, 109, 122, 123
Jesness, C. F., 82–83, 93, 123
Jessor, R., 8, 123,
Jessor, S. L., 8, 123
Jones, S. E., 32, 119

Kaemmer, B., 82, 118
Kagan, N., 73, 118
Kalas, R., 62, 119
Kamphus, R. W., 59, 60, 126
Kauffman, J. M., 61–62, 121
Kaufman, A. S., 44, 50–51, 123
Kaufman, N. L., 50–51, 123
Kazdin, A. E., 12, 63, 64, 87, 88, 99, 106, 107, 123
Keenan, K., 107, 124
Keyser, D. J., 42, 103, 123
Kiessling, J. J., 92, 117
Klaric, S. H., 62, 119
Kline, R. B., 123
Klinnert, M., 72, 125
Knight, R. A., 109, 123
Knowles, B. A., 119
Koepke, T., 72, 126
Kolb, B., 49, 123
Kolko, D. J., 87, 88, 123
Kopelman, F., 24, 119
Kravitz, D. A., 64, 123
Krechevsky, M., 120
Krisberg, B., 79, 85, 87, 100, 128

Lacher, D. O., 123
Lahey, B. B., 60, 107, 124, 128
Lanyon, R., 101, 123
Last, C. G., 63, 123
L'Abate, L., 70, 75–76, 123
Lavoie, Y., 71, 125
Le Blanc, B., 4, 8, 123
LeCroy, C. W., 10, 23, 52, 66, 69, 87, 88, 94, 95, 106, 117, 118
Leipciger, M., 64, 65, 120
Leschied, A. W., 12, 13, 24, 26–27, 56, 69, 80, 83–84, 92, 93, 104, 109, 117, 122, 123, 127
Lezak, M. D., 49, 124
Lilienfield, S. O., 60, 128
Lipsey, M. W., 106, 124
Loeber, R., 12, 37, 69, 99, 105, 106, 107, 124, 127
Luthar, S. S., 13, 124

MacDonald III, A. W., 105, 118
Mak, A. S., 60, 61, 124

Mann, B. J., 69, 75, 118
Markwart, A., 5, 6, 40–41, 69, 119, 124
Marsh, H. W., 58, 124
Marston, N. C., 59, 124
Mash, E. J., 55, 64, 124
Matatazzo, J. D., 35, 41, 101, 124
McBurnett, K., 88, 120
McConaughy, S. H., 60, 63, 104, 117, 124
McDermott, P. A., 19, 20, 59, 124
McFall, R. M., 63–64, 120
McKnew, D., 63, 122
McReynolds, P., 81, 124
Meagher, R. B., 56, 57, 125
Meehl, P. E., 25, 119
Megargee, E. I., 79, 81, 124
Melton, G. B., 24, 35, 41, 53, 75, 103, 121, 125
Menard, S., 61, 120
Menzies, R. J., 37, 121
Messick, S., 33, 34, 125
Meyer, R. G., 55, 125
Miller, J. Y., 12, 106, 121
Miller, R. D., 35, 41, 53, 121
Millon, T., 56, 57, 125, 128
Mitchell, C. N., 17, 21, 24, 35, 41, 102, 126
Moos, B., 70, 71, 125
Moos, R. H., 70, 71, 74, 84, 118, 125
Morris, A., 8, 125
Moye, A., 71, 72, 126
Moyer, S., 24, 119
Mrazek, D. A., 72, 125
Mrazek, P., 72, 125
Mulvey, E. P., 17, 21, 24, 106, 127, 128
Murphy, K. R., 62, 125

Nagy, T. F., 32, 119
Neuberger, A. R., 25–26, 120
Newman, J. P., 88, 121
Niarhos, F. J., 24, 125
Novy, D., 73, 118
Noy, J. E., 83, 122

Ogloff, J. R. P., 108, 126
O'Brien, B. S., 90, 120

O'Brien, J. D., 62, 63, 81, 88, 121
O'Neill, R., 58, 124
Okagaki, L., 46–47, 120
Olson, D. H., 71, 125
Onek, D., 79, 85, 87, 100, 128
Ouimet, M., 8, 123
Overall, J. E., 59, 125

Palmer, T., 79, 106, 125
Partner, J., 71, 125
Patterson, G. R., 71, 99–100, 105, 124, 125
Patton, J. H., 127
Perlmutter, B. F., 70, 127
Peterson, D. R., 59, 72, 99, 126
Petrila, J., 24, 35, 41, 53, 103, 125
Pfefferbaum, B., 59, 125
Piacentini, J., 62, 63, 105, 127
Poythress, N. G., 24, 35, 41, 53, 103, 125
Pratt, J., 3, 4, 125
Prentky, R., 109, 124

Quay, H. C., 59, 72, 79, 81, 84, 99, 107, 125, 126

Ramsey, E., 99, 125
Raven, J., 46, 126
Raven, J. C., 46, 126
Realmuto, G. M., 105, 118
Reddon, J. R., 122
Regier, D., 63, 105, 127
Reid, J. B., 99–10, 125
Reid, S. A., 3, 71, 126
Reitan, R. M., 48, 126
Reitsma-Street, M., 3, 80, 83–84, 93, 109, 126
Renzulli, J. S., 58, 122
Reppucci, N. D., 21, 106, 125, 127, 128
Reynolds, C. R., 59, 60, 126
Rigby, K., 64, 126
Robblee, M. A., 92, 117
Robin, A. L., 71, 72, 126
Robinson, D., 92, 117
Roehling, P. V., 71, 126

Roesch, R., 92, 108, 126
Rogers, J. M., 17, 21, 21, 24, 35, 41, 53, 102, 128
Rogers, R., 53, 126
Rosenthal, L., 63–64, 120
Rosser, M. E., 83, 122
Rotatori, A. F., 58, 126
Routh, D. K., 24, 81, 125, 126
Rutter, M., 13, 126

Sadoff, R.L., 35, 41, 53, 121
Sas, L., 56, 104, 122
Sattler, J. M., 42, 44, 48, 49, 55, 61–62, 64, 81, 126
Saunders, R., 92, 117
Sbordone, R. J., 49, 126
Schaefer, E., 72, 126
Schissel, B., 24, 26, 126
Schluderman, E., 72, 126, 127
Schluderman, S., 72, 126, 127
Schlundt, D. G., 63–64, 120
Schoenwald, S. K., 75, 121
Schwab-Stone, M., 62, 63, 105, 127
Sellin, T., 20, 127
Shaffer, D., 62, 63, 105, 127
Shapiro, S. K., 81, 126
Shaw, M. W., 64, 127
Sheu, W. J., 61, 127
Shields, I. W., 64, 65, 105, 127
Shutt, R., 24, 119
Siassi, I., 62, 127
Silvaroli, N. J., 47, 127
Simourd, D. J., 65, 92, 127
Skinner, H. A., 61, 127
Slobogin, C., 24, 35, 41, 53, 103, 125
Smiley, W. C ., 122
Smith, L. A., 75, 121
Smitherman, H. W., 65, 118
Snow, R. E., 76, 127
Sorensen, D. E., 104, 118
Sparrow, S. S., 61, 62, 127
Stanford, M. S., 88, 127
Sternberg, R., 46, 120, 127
Stott, D. H., 59, 124
Stouthamer-Loeber, M., 12, 69, 99, 106, 124
Straus, M. A., 70, 127
Strayhorn, J.M., 72, 127

Stylianos, S., 21, 128
Sweetland, R. C., 42, 103, 123

Tarter, R. E., 61, 127
Tate, D. C., 106, 127
Tellegen, R. P., 82, 118
Tennenbaum, D. L., 70, 122
Terdal, L. G., 55, 64, 124
Thomas, C. W., 24, 107, 124, 127
Thornberry, T. P., 106, 127
Tomkins, A., 26, 121
Touliatos, J., 70, 127
Tremblay, R. E., 8, 106, 123, 127
Trevethan, S. D., 90, 128
Turnbull, S. D., 4, 5, 24, 25, 119
Tutt, N., 16, 120

Utada, A., 63–64, 120

Valcuikas, J. A., 49, 128
Vaneziano, C., 81, 128
Vaneziano, L., 81, 128
Van Voorhis, P., 79, 128
Vold, G., 128

Waldman, I. D., 60, 107, 128
Walker, L. J., 90, 128
Warren, M. Q., 80, 82, 83, 128
Weatherman, R. F., 62, 118
Webster, C. D., 21, 37, 92, 121, 128
Wechsler, D., 30, 44, 48–49, 98, 128
Wedge, R.F., 93, 123
Weidman, C. S., 72, 127
Weinberger, D. A., 72, 99–100, 120
Weisstub, D., 92, 128
Werry, J. S., 63, 128
West, D., 92, 117
Wheatt, T., 62, 122
Whishaw, I. Q., 49, 123
Whitehall, G. C., 64, 65, 105, 127

Wiebush, R. G., 79, 85, 87, 100, 128
Williams, C. L., 82, 118
Williams, J., 88, 127
Williams, R. A., 75, 118
Wilson, D. B., 106, 124
Wolfgang, M. E., 20, 127
Wolfson, D., 48, 126
Woodcock, R. W., 62, 118
Woodward, M. J., 56, 128
Woolard, J. L., 21, 128
Wooton, J. M., 88, 120
Wormith, J. S., 104, 128
Wright, K. N., 74, 128
Wright, M., 64, 127

Yoshikawa, H., 69, 106, 107, 128
Young, J. G., 62, 63, 81, 85, 121
Young, W., 85, 120
Yung, B., 109, 121

Zager, L. D., 81, 109, 128

Subject Index

Academic achievement, measures of, 50–51; *see also specific tests*
    juvenile justice system, role in, 51–53
Adaptive functioning, measures of, 61–62
Adjudication, 17
Adolescent Drug Abuse Diagnosis Interview, 63
Adolescent Problem Inventory, 63–64
Aggravating factors, judgments about youth and, 20–21, 66
American Educational Research Association, 31
American Psychological Association, 31
Antisocial behavior, measures of, 60–61
Aptitude, assessment measures; *see also specific tests*
    assessment measures, 43–50
    cognitive ability, tests of, 43–47
    juvenile justice system, role in, 51–53
    neuropsychological assessments, 48–49
    specific aptitudes, measures of, 47–48
    vocational aptitude and interest tests, 49–50
Aptitude attributes
    criminal behavior, causal variable, 9
Arizona Juvenile Risk Assessment Form, 88, 94–95
Armed Services Vocational Aptitude Battery, 50
Assessments, psychological: *see* Psychological assessments, role in decision process
Assessment of Children (third edition, revised), 42
Associates
    antisocial, criminal behavior and, 9, 12
    measures of associations, 73–74
Attention-Deficit/Hyperactivity Disorder, 34–35, 52, 80
Attitudes
    criminal behavior and, 9
    measures of: *see* Personality, attitudes, and behaviors, assessment of

Basic Personality Inventory, 56, 66, 104, 107
Behavioral history, criminal behavior and, 9

Behaviorally based diagnostic systems, 84, 93–94
Behavioral ratings and checklists, 59–62; *see also* Personality, attitudes, and behaviors, assessment of
    adaptive functioning, 61–62
    antisocial behavior, 60–61
    emotional competence, 59–60
    self-destructive behavior, 60–61
    social competence, 59–60
Behavior Assessment System for Children, 60
Behavior Problem Checklist, 60
Beliefs
    criminal behavior and, 9
    measures of, 64–65
Bennett Mechanical Comprehension Test, 50
Bennett's Self-Esteem Scale, 104
BPI: *see* Basic Personality Inventory
Brain damage or dysfunction, neuropsychological assessments, 48–49
Broad based risk instruments of diagnosis, 87, 94–95

Canada, *see also specific topics throughout this index*; Young Offenders Act of Canada
    Criminal Code s. 515(10), 22
CAS: *see* Child Assessment Schedule
Case classification, risk and, 10t
Child Assessment Schedule, 62–63
Child Behavior Checklist, 60, 72, 73
Child Behavior Checklist-Teacher Report Form, 60
Children's Apperception Test, 64
Children's Report of Parental Behavior, 72
Child welfare model of juvenile justice
    criminogenic need, judgment regarding, 22
    described, 4, 7
    environmental factors, assessment of, 69

Child welfare model of juvenile justice (*cont.*)
General Personality and Social Psychological Model of Criminal Conduct and, 13, 69
orientation of, 7
Classifications systems: *see* Diagnostic and classification systems
Classroom Observation Code, 64
Classroom Reading Inventory, 47–48
Clinical Interview for Children, 60
CLMM: *see* Conceptual Level Matching Model
Cognitive ability, tests of, 43–47; *see also specific tests*
general intelligence tests, 44t
group intelligence tests, 44t, 45–46
individual intelligence tests, 44t, 45
juvenile justice system, role in, 52
nonverbal or performance intelligence tests, 44t, 46
College of Psychologists of Ontario, 32
Colorado Security Placement Instrument, 85, 86t
Community-Oriented Programs Environment Scale, 74, 76
Competence Assessment for Standing Trial for Defendants with Mental Retardation, 92
Competency to Stand Trial Assessment Instrument, 92
Computer-aided scoring of assessments, 101
Conceptual background, 1–13
juvenile justice, models of, 7–8
Conceptual Level Matching Model, 83–84, 93–94
Conduct disorder, 35, 80
Consistency, psychological assessments, 98, 103
Construct development, research recommendations, 107–108
Construct validity, psychological assessments, 34–35, 37
Content validity, psychological assessments, 34
Contingency tables, 36–37
Corporatist model of juvenile justice, 3f
criminogenic need, judgment regarding, 22
described, 4–5
Correctional environments, measures of, 74–77
Correctional Institutions Environmental Scale, 74, 76–77, 84
Correctional Program Assessment Inventory, 74

Crime control model of juvenile justice, 3f
described, 6–7
mitigating and aggravating factors, 20
risk assessment and, 22
seriousness of offense and, 19
Criminal behavior, theories of, 8t; *see also* General Personality and Social Psychological Model of Criminal Conduct
aptitude attributes, 9
associates, antisocial, as causal factor, 9, 12
attitudinal variables, 9
behavioral history as causal variable, 9
education, effect of, 10
family relationships and, 12
personality attributes, 9
risk factors, 10
values and beliefs, 9
Criminal Sentiments Scale, 65
Criminogenic need, judgments about youth regarding, 22–23, 52
Criminological processes, research recommendations, 106–107
Criterion validity, psychological assessments, 35–36
CTPI-Level Interview, 82

Decision making, 15–27
forensic, 15–18
inappropriate decisions, 1–2, 15
inconsistency in applying rules, 2, 25–27
invalid decisions, 1–2, 15, 25–27
judgments about youth and their circumstances, 18–24
juvenile justice system, within, 15–27
processes, 24–27
psychological assessments, role of: *see* Psychological assessments, role in decision process
Delinquency, theories of, 7–8
Diagnostic and classification systems, 79–95
behaviorally based diagnostic systems, 84, 93–94
broad-based risk instruments, 87, 94–95
juvenile justice systems, role in, 93–95
offense-based risk systems, 84–87, 94
personality-based systems, 79–84, 93–94
risk/need instruments, 87, 91t, 94–95
Diagnostic and Statistical Manual of Mental Disorders, Third Edition, Revised, 62

Diagnostic and Statistical Manual of Mental Disorders, Fourth Edition, 62, 66
criticisms of, 81
described, 80–81
juvenile justice systems, role in, 93–94
Diagnostic Interview Schedule for Children and Adolescents, 62
Direct Observation Form, 60, 64
Disposition, forensic decision making, 18
Disruptive Behavior Disorder, 80
DSM-III-R: *see Diagnostic and Statistical Manual of Mental Disorders*, Third Edition, Revised
DSM-IV: *see Diagnostic and Statistical Manual of Mental Disorders*, Fourth Edition
Dynamic predictive validity, psychological assessments, 37
personality tests, 58

Education
attitudes toward, measures of, 73t
criminal behavior and, 10
Emotional competence, ratings of, 59–60
Environmental factors, assessment of, 69–77; *see also specific tests and scales*
correctional environments, measures of, 74–77
educational attitudes, 73t
family functioning, measures of, 70 72, 75 76
juvenile justice systems, role in, 75–77
parenting, measures of, 70–72, 75–76
school performance and adjustment, measures of, 72–73
therapeutic environments, measures of, 74–77
Evaluation of psychological assessment instruments, 30–38
contingency tables, 36–37
definition of terms, 33t
reliability, defined, 33
terminology, 32–38
validity, defined, 33–37
Expertise, 101–102

Family
criminal behavior and family relationships, 12
delinquency, family factors, 99–100
functioning, measures of, 70–72, 75–76

Family Environment Scale, 70–71
subscales, 71t
Family Events Checklist, 99
Federal Bureau of Investigation (FBI) Violent Crime Index, 20
Firesetting Risk Interview, 88
Fitness Interview Test, 92
Forensic decision making, 15–18; *see also* Personality, attitudes, and behaviors, assessment of; Psychological assessments, role in decision process
adjudication, 17
disposition, 18
intake/preadjudicatory processing, 17
major statutory areas within juvenile justice system, 16t, 18
police investigations/processing, 16–17

General Personality and Social Psychological Model of Criminal Conduct, 8, 10
assessing responsivity, 66
broad-based risk/need instruments and, 95
cognitive ability, importance of, 52
criminogenic need, judgment regarding, 22
environmental factors, assessment of, 69
implications of, 15
principles of, 11t, 12
risk factors, 11t
targets of change, 11t
Group intelligence tests, 44t, 45–46

Halstead-Reitan Neuropsychological Test Battery for Older Children, 48–49
Hare Psychopathology Checklist, 30
Hyperactivity, 35

I-Level: *see* Interpersonal Maturity Level Classification System
Inappropriate decisions: *see* Decision making
Inconsistency, decision making and application of rules, 2, 25–27
Incremental predictive validity, psychological assessments, 37
Individual intelligence tests, 44t
limitations, 45
Instrument development, research recommendations, 108–109
Intake assessment battery, model, 105t
Intake/preadjudicatory processing, 17

Intelligence tests
 group intelligence tests, 44t, 45–46
 individual intelligence tests, 44t, 45
 juvenile justice system, role in, 52
 nonverbal or performance tests, 44t, 46
 types of, 44t
Interpersonal Maturity Level Classification
 System, 82–83, 93
Intervention
 aptitude and achievement tests, role in assessments, 52
 effectiveness, research recommendations,
  107
 personality tests and, 93
Interview for Antisocial Behavior, 64
Interview schedules, 62–64, 63t
Invalid decisions: *see* Decision making
IQ tests: *see* Intelligence tests

Jackson Vocational Interest Survey, 49
Jesness Inventory, 56, 82–83
Judgments about youth and their circumstances
 aggravating factors, 20–21, 66
 criminogenic need, 22–23, 52
 maturity level, 21, 41
 mental illness, 21
 mitigating factors, 20–21, 66
 rehabilitation, possibility of, 22–23
 responsivity, 24, 66–67
 risk level, assessment of, 21–22, 52
 seriousness of offense, 18–24
 treatment, amenability to, 23–24
Justice: *see* Juvenile justice, models of
Justice model of juvenile justice, 3f
 described, 5–7
 risk assessment and, 22
 seriousness of offense and, 19
Juvenile justice, models of, 2–7
 child welfare model, 4, 7, 13, 22, 69
 continuum of, 3f
 corporatist model, 3f, 4–5, 22
 crime control model, 3f, 6, 19–20, 22
 justice model, 3f, 5–7, 19, 22
 modified justice model, 3f, 5, 7, 13, 19, 22
 purposes of judicial dispositions, 6–7
 welfare model, 3f
Juvenile justice systems, generally: *see specific
 topic*

Kaufman Test of Educational Achievement,
 50

Labeling, psychological assessment and, 40–41
Level of Service Inventory, 90
LSI: *see* Level of Service Inventory

MAPI: *see* Millon Adolescent Personality In-
 ventory
Maturity of youth, judgments and, 21, 41
Mental illness of youth, judgment and, 21
Mental Measurements Yearbook, 55, 103
Millon Adolescent Personality Inventory, 56,
 57t, 80
Minnesota Multiphasic Inventory–2, 82, 109
Minnesota Multiphasic Inventory–Adolescent,
 56
 aggravating conditions, information on, 66
 applications of, 82
 DSM-IV diagnostic categories and, 80
 intervention decisions and, 93
Minnesota Multiphasic Inventory
 background, 1
 described, 81–82
Mitigating factors, judgments about youth and,
 20–21, 66
MMPI: *see* Minnesota Multiphasic Inventory
MMPI–2: *see* Minnesota Multiphasic Inventory–2
MMPI–A: *see* Minnesota Multiphasic Inventory–Adolescent
Modified justice model of juvenile justice, 3f
 criminogenic need, judgment regarding, 22
 described, 5
 General Personality and Social Psychological Model of Criminal Conduct and,
  13
 orientation of, 7
 risk assessment and, 22
 seriousness of defense and, 19
Multidimensional Self-Concept Scale, 58

National Council on Measurement in Education, 31
Need
 criminogenic, judgments about youth regarding, 22–23, 52
 principle of, 11t, 12
 risk/need instruments of diagnosis, 87, 91t,
  94–95
Neuropsychological assessments, 48–49
Nonverbal or performance intelligence tests,
 44t, 46
North Dakota Risk Assessment Instrument, 85

Offense-based risk systems of diagnosis, 84–87
  juvenile justice system, role in, 94

Paragraph Completion Method, 83
Parenting, measures of, 70–72, 75–76
Parenting Risk Scale, 71
PCL–R: *see* Psychopathology Checklist–Revised
Peer groups
  antisocial associates, criminal behavior and, 9, 12
  measures of associations, 73–74
Personality, attitudes, and behaviors, assessment of, 55–67; *see also specific tests and scales*
  attitudes, measures of, 64–65
  behavioral ratings and checklists, 59–62
  beliefs, measures of, 64–65
  interview schedules, 62–64
  juvenile justice system, role of measures in, 65–67
  personality tests, 55–58
  projective instruments, 64
  structured observation schedules, 64
  values, measures of, 64–65
Personality attributes
  criminal behavior, causal variable, 9
Personality-based diagnostic systems, 79–84, 93–94; *see also specific tests and scales*
  behaviorally based systems, 84
  DSM-IV, 80–81
Personality tests, 55–58
  validity, 57–58
Personnel, disposition decisions and, 18
Police investigations/processing, 16–17
Practitioners, recommendations in use of psychological assessments
  assessment batteries, formation of, 103–104, 105t
  expertise, role of, 101–102
  selection of instruments, 102–105
Predictive validity, psychological assessments, 35
Pride in Delinquency Scale, 65
Prison Environment Inventory, 74, 76–77, 84
Professional override principle, 12
Professional standards
  psychological assessments, evaluation, 31–32
Projective instruments, 64

Psychological assessments, role in decision process, 29–42; *see also* Forensic decision making; *specific tests and scales*
  assessment batteries, formation of, 103–104, 105t
  cautions, 42
  clarity, 103
  computer-aided scoring, 101
  consensus, lack of, 40
  consistency, 98, 103
  constructs
    development, research recommendations, 107–108
    explicitness of, 98–99
  contingency tables, 36–37
  definition of terms, 33t
  drawbacks of psychological assessments, 39–41
  efficiency of system, 100
  evaluation of instruments, 30–38, 100
  instrument development, research recommendations, 108–109
  instruments and procedures, major types of, 29–30
  labeling, dangers of, 40–41
  positive contributions of, 97–100
  practitioners, recommendations for, 100–105
  professional standards, 31–32
  relevance, importance of, 37–38
  reliability, defined, 33
  research recommendations, 105–109
  selection of instruments, 102–105
  standardized assessments, potential strengths of, 38–39
  substantive findings, access to, 99–100
  terminology for evaluating, 32–38
  tools, availability of, 97–98
  validity, definitions, 33–37
Psychopathology Checklist, 64, 66, 101
Psychopathology Checklist–Revised, 88–90, 95

Quick Neurological Screening Test, 49

Raven's Progressive Matrices, 46
RBPC: *see* Revised Behavior Problem Checklist
Rehabilitation, judgments about youth regarding possibility of, 22–23
Reliability, defined, 33

Research recommendations, psychological assessments
  construct development, 107–108
  criminological processes, 106–107
  instrument development, 108–109
Responsivity
  assessment of, 66–67
  description of principle of, 12
  judgments regarding, 24
Revised Behavior Problem Checklist
  described, 59
  juvenile justice systems, role in, 66
  positive contributions of, 99
  school performance and adjustment, measure of, 72
Revised Diagnostic Interview Schedule for Children, 62
Risk
  achievement tests, relevance to judgments on risk levels, 52
  aptitude tests, relevance to judgments on risk levels, 52
  assessment regarding level of, 21–22, 52, 66
  broad-based risk instruments of diagnosis, 87, 94–95
  case classification and, 10t
  offense-based risk systems of diagnosis, 84–87
  risk/need instruments of diagnosis, 87, 91t, 94–95
Rorschach test, 64

Salient Factor Score Index, 85
School performance and adjustment, measures of, 72–73
Self-concept, measures of, 58
Self-Description Questionnaire, 58
Self-destructive behavior, measures of, 60–61
Self-esteem, measures of, 58, 104
Self-Reported Delinquency Scale, 60
Self-reporting, self-destructive behaviors, 60, 61t
Semistructured Clinical Interview for Children, 63–64
Sentencing Factors Inventory, 92
Seriousness of offense, decision making and, 19–20
Shipley Institute of Living Scale, 45
Singapore, juvenile justice system in, 6
Social and emotional competence, ratings of, 59–60
Social Climate Scales, 74

Specialized Aptitude Test, 47
Standardized psychological assessments: see Psychological assessments, role in decision process
Standards for Educational and Psychological Testing (American Psychological Association), 42, 101
  described, 31–32
  terminology for evaluation, 32
Structured observation schedules, 64
Student Attitude Measure, 73
Symptom Complex Scales of the CAS, 63

Test Critiques, 42, 55, 103
Test of Auditory Comprehension of Language–Revised, 47
Theoretical background, 1–13
  contemporary psychological perspective, 8–13
  criminal behavior, major theories of, 8t
  delinquency, theories of, 7–8
  juvenile justice, models of, 7–8
Theory of Multiple Intelligences (Gardner), 46–47
Therapeutic environments, measures of, 74–77
Treatment, judgments regarding amenability to, 23–24
Triarchic Theory of Intelligence, 46
The 12th Mental Measurements Yearbook, 42

United Kingdom, juvenile justice systems: see specific topics throughout this index
United States, juvenile justice systems: see specific topics throughout this index
United States Parole Commission, 85
U.S. Department of Defense, 50

Validity
  construct validity, 34–35, 37
  content validity, 34
  criterion validity, 35–36
  dynamic predictive validity, 37, 58
  incremental predictive validity, 37
  invalid decisions: see Decision making
  personality tests, 57–58
  predictive validity, 35
  psychological assessments, defined for purposes of, 33–37
Values
  criminal behavior and, 9
  measures of, 64–65

Vineland Adaptive Behavior Scales, 61
Violent Crime Index of FBI, 20
Vocational aptitude and interest tests, 49–50

Wechsler Adult Intelligence Scale–Revised, 30
Wechsler Intelligence Scale for Children, 44,
    98, 101
Weinberger Parenting Inventory, 99–100
Welfare model of juvenile justice, 3f
WISC-III: *see* Wechsler Intelligence Scale for
    Children

Wisconsin Juvenile Probation and Aftercare As-
    sessment Form, 87–88

YLS/CMI: *see* Youth Level of Service/Case
    Management Inventory
Young Offenders Act of Canada, 51
    decision making and application of rules, 26
    disposition and, 18
Youth Level of Service/Case Management In-
    ventory, 90–92, 95, 98, 101
Youth Self-Report Inventory, 60